W9-CCT-261

"*End Medical Debt* is special because it advocates for systemic change, while providing tactical solutions for Americans facing the devastating burden of medical debt now. Tens of millions of Americans live paycheck-to-paycheck. They feel completely shut out of our financial system. *End Medical Debt* and RIP Medical Debt's mission empowers working-class families to find ways to alleviate this undue burden. Equally important, it gives them hope for a new version of the American medical system — one that's designed to work for them, rather than against them."

Rohan Pavluri
CEO, Upsolve. TED Talk

"More and more Americans are compounding their serious health issues with unprecedented and unmanageable medical debt. Meanwhile, a small self-appointed group of experts from the world of healthcare finance are seeking solutions for a broken system. Where there are no acceptable answers yet, people are creating them. Jerry Ashton, Robert Goff and Craig Antico are putting lifetimes of experience to work in *End Medical Debt* to spread the word that medical debt is a personal and national crisis. More so, they are offering answers that are gaining national attention."

Kevin A. Cahill
New York State Assemblyman (District 103)
Chair, Assembly Committee on Insurance

"*End Medical Debt* is exactly what is needed to jumpstart the much-needed national discussion about our current dysfunctional for-profit health care system, and what to do about it, so patients like me don't have to experience the financial and personal hardships caused by medical debt. We are a forgotten, disposable, invisible universe of people. There are millions of us. This book explains with passion and honesty the nightmare of medical debt."

Joel R. Segal
Former senior legislative assistant, U.S. Congress (2000 to 2019),
Co-author, HR 676: "Expanded and Improved Medicare For All"

"The three authors, who assist people with medical debt, write about the medical crisis of this country in all its forms. They tackle sound and logical solutions that could be instituted by politicians, doctors, pharmaceuticals and average citizens. *End Medical Debt* is a valuable resource that should be read by every American citizen to make our health care system the best it can be in the world."

Midwest Review of Books

"*End Medical Debt* does more than describe the unsustainable structure of our current health care system. The book demonstrates what was always the solution: People helping people, voluntarily and without coercion. The current healthcare system has created a debt-enslaved class with few options. Necessity will produce many solutions, but in the meantime, the book offers us hope from those willing and able to pay forward their success. Humanity at its best.

Ernest Hancock
Publisher, FreedomsPhoenix

"America spends more on medical care than any other country, and the resulting medical debt is our nation's primary reason for bankruptcy and financial ruin. I've seen the impact. *End Medical Debt* offers clear answers on what people can do for themselves and society to end this scourge."

Ed Asner
Actor, Activist

"Ashton, Antico and Goff are modern day monetary musketeers, slaying the medical debt endured by millions of Americans. Their book on our dysfunctional and unsustainable medical landscape is a catalyst to enhance our understanding and eventual repair of that landscape. *End Medical Debt* demonstrates Americans can come together from across diverse viewpoints and find agreement."

Marion Mass, MD
Pediatrician, cofounder, Free2Care

END
MEDICAL
DEBT

*Of all the forms of inequality,
injustice in health is the most
shocking and inhumane.*

— MARTIN LUTHER KING, JR.

END MEDICAL DEBT

Curing America's Healthcare Crisis

Jerry Ashton
Robert E. Goff
Craig Antico

Edited by Judah Freed

HOKU HOUSE

END MEDICAL DEBT
Curing America's Healthcare Crisis

Book Website: EndMedicalDebt.com
Publisher Website: HokuHouse.com

Published by Hoku House, Denver, Colorado
    Editor, Cover & Book Designer: Judah Freed

Printed in the United States of America.
Electronic book in epub format.

Cloth Hardcover:	ISBN-13: 978-1-7373985-1-6
Trade Softcover:	ISBN-13: 978-1-7373985-0-9
eBook:	ISBN-13: 978-1-7373985-2-3

Please contact the publisher at HokuHouse.com for special orders.

First edition published in December 2018.
Second revised edition published in October 2021

ALL author royalties donated for medical debt forgiveness.

Cataloging-in-Publication Data:

Ashton, Jerry, 1937 —
Goff, Robert E., 1952 —
Antico, Craig, 1961 —

    END MEDICAL DEBT
    Curing America's Healthcare Crisis

280 pages with 13 Chapters, Preface, Introduction.

    1. Contemporary Affairs. 2. Personal Finance.
    3. Politics/Government. 4. Health 5. Economics.

Praise for END MEDICAL DEBT

"If you want to read a book about how the healthcare system in the world's richest country can fail so many — including millions of middle-class Americans who have what they believe is good health insurance — that book is *End Medical Debt*. The authors, who willed RIP Medical Debt into existence, have written one of the best books I've come across that explains how the U.S. healthcare system became a voracious monster, and the steps we can take, individually and collectively, to keep it from devouring us all."

Wendell Potter
President, Center for Health and Democracy

"We need *sunshine* and *transparency* in healthcare, and this book by Jerry Ashton, Craig Antico and Robert Goff does a great job at throwing open those windows and letting those clear rays shine through. The Covid recovery edition of *End Medical Debt* breaks down the critical issues in a way that's easy to understand. As a practicing physician involved in grassroots healthcare advocacy, it's refreshing to have these three men in our corner."

Marlene Wust-Smith, MD
Founder and Publisher, Physician Outlook Magazine

"*End Medical Debt* confronts an important, sad truth: No one asks to be sick. It's hard enough being poor; it's hard enough being sick. But being poor and sick becomes a death sentence for some, a life sentence of indentured servitude for others. The bills are almost beyond belief. I went into the hospital overnight with chest pains, and the hospital bill was $25,000. It's time to lift this yoke off the necks of the most vulnerable and defenseless members of society."

Alan Grayson
Former U.S. Congressman (D-FL)

"*End Medical Debt* is a must-read for anyone who wants a complete understanding of the how and why of our arcane healthcare system. and for anyone who wants to understand what are our options."

Egberto Willies
Producer and Host, Politics Done Right

"No one chooses a life threatening illness, and no one should have to lose almost everything to pay for the treatment they need to save their lives or the lives of their loved ones. How can a system that pays more per patient than any other country have such dismal health outcomes? While we await long overdue systemic changes in America's healthcare industry, we can be inspired to act on the practical, humane solutions served up by authors Jerry Ashton, Robert Goff and Craig Antico in *End Medical Debt*."

Nancy A. Niparko, MD
Child Neurologist

"*End Medical Debt* is a must read that reveals the truth about the U.S. public health system. Medical debt and Covid-19 resurgences are the inevitable outcomes of a system that is killing America."

Katherine Sullivan
Founder, 360 Wellness Solutions

"As an entrepreneur committed to reducing the burden that poverty creates for millions of Americans, I have heard many pitches directed toward helping hospitals and healthcare providers, increase revenue without regard or concern for the healthcare consumers. For this reason, I am inspired by the collective efforts of the diverse team writing *End Medical Debt.*

Ed Connors
CEO/President, Heudia Health

"Give me your tired, your poor, your huddled masses, but be well insured! The medical industrial Sick Complex accepts nothing less. *End Medical Debt* illustrates that each and every one of us is a car accident or cancer diagnosis away from significant financial problems. We are better than this."

Doug Aldeen
ERISA Health Care Attorney
[Employee Retirement Income Security Act]

Dedication

For all who struggle with medical debt,
and for all who care to abolish it.

We must not let our rulers
load us with perpetual debt.

— THOMAS JEFFERSON

END MEDICAL DEBT

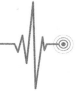

Table of Contents

About the Book

Judah Freed, Editor

Welcome to the revised and expanded Covid recovery edition of *End Medical Debt*, a #1 bestseller on Amazon and Barnes & Noble for health policy books, top 100 for personal finance, after coverage on *PBS NewsHour, Associated Press* and elsewhere.

End Medical Debt offers the big picture of our healthcare system with realistic insights on our personal and national solutions.

The three authors are insiders of debt collections and healthcare administration. Instead of collecting unpayable bills, in 2014 they co-founded RIP Medical Debt, a charity that locates, buys and forgives the medical bills causing hardship for Americans. RIP has abolished $5 billion in medical debt, so far. For scale, *The New York Times* in July 2021 reported the current U.S. medical debt is $140 billion.

This update aims to help recovery from Covid-19 (SARS-CoV-2) and variants. The economy entered recession after the public health shutdowns. Due to the very nature of health care delivery in America, millions of people are getting medical bills they cannot pay.

The authors view debt forgiveness as necessary but insufficient, an interim solution until we agree on a better financial structure for the U.S. healthcare system. Legislation pending in Congress could be a healthy step in that direction, but it's not a cure.

The authors bring deep expertise to the issues of medical debt. **Jerry Ashton** has 40 years of experience in credit and collections. **Robert E. Goff** has retired from 45 years in healthcare management. **Craig Antico** has 30 years in collections, debt buying, outsourcing. Their politics vary widely. Jerry is progressive. Robert is moderate. Craig is conservative. Together their energies are dynamic.

Incorporating the RIP charity in 2014, Craig was the CEO, Jerry was the Executive VP, and Robert was the founding board member. Robert and Jerry wrote a book together, *The Patient, The Doctor and The Bill Collector,* which Hoku House published in January 2016. That book led to RIP being on HBO's John Oliver show.

"The John Oliver Effect," let RIP hire a team for donations and debt buying. RIP hired me as consultant to do the website and public relations, initially. The growth by 2020 let RIP hire NYC nonprofits leader Allison Sesso as the Executive Director. Jerry and Robert now serve on the board, where Craig is emeritus.

After Oliver, Jerry wanted to write a new book. Robert wanted to speak more openly than he could when still a healthcare administrator. Craig felt a passion to express his own thoughts. I agreed to be editor and publisher. Our collaboration created the 2018 edition of *End Medical Debt.* This 2021 edition updates their facts, deepens their insights, and adds a conversation among the authors.

Each author wrote his chapters without seeing the others' work, waiting to read the full book until my layout was complete, then we all tweaked the text. The views of each author are his own. Balancing their distinct voices has been my distinct pleasure as editor.

NOTE: Hoku House pays the authors *85 percent* of all the book revenues (opposite of most book deals where authors get a pittance). ***The authors donate ALL of their royalties to forgive medical debt.*** Each book sold abolishes about $500 in unpayable medical bills.

— JF

Acknowledgments

The creators of *End Medical Debt* have great people to thank for help in producing this book. We each speak in turn:

Jerry Ashton: My fullest expression of gratitude goes to my co-authors and the publisher, without whose efforts this book and the success of RIP Medical Debt would not have happened. First in line after them is my wife, Kate Coburn, and my wonderful daughters, Andrea and Alexandra, for their unfailing support — my anchor in every storm. The magnetic center of influence in my personal and professional growth has been Occupy Wall Street and my experience with its "Rolling Jubilee" experiment in debt forgiveness, which inspired our charity. Occupy was a petri dish for ideas and solutions to develop and mature, RIP is one of them. Here's to all you Occupiers, past and present, who caused me to be aware and then motivated me to put that awareness into responsible action.

Robert E. Goff: My contributions to the book would not be possible without immersion for over 45 years in the American health-care system. Nearly 20 years with the University Physicians Network gave me insights to practitioners of the art and science of medical practice with care and compassion. Such leaders as doctors Stuart Garay, Sol Zimmerman and Paula Marchetta are examples. I'm grateful for a decade of collaboration with Edward Ullman to create and operate one of New York's earliest HMOs, trying to offer both quality and affordability in health care coverage. The variety of roles in my career contributed different perspectives. My wife Jinny and son Blake's experience as healthcare consumers kept me grounded in the actual patient experience within the disjointed healthcare non-system. I also want to acknowledge my co-authors, Jerry Ashton and Craig Antico, for their energy and creativity in forming RIP Medical Debt, whose social mission this book seeks to support.

Craig Antico: I wish to thank: Jerry Ashton, progressive activist and gadfly (my balance) turned partner, friend and wise mentor; you haven't changed; but, thanks to you, I have. Jessica, spouse of great sacrifice, giver, cheerleader, loyal best friend, an intelligent, caring, conservative influence. My uniquely caring sons Erik, Clark, Alex, Connor, and Chad. My optimistic and well-read father, Al. Mother Barbara never gave up on me! Andy Goldstone, using TransUnion health data through RIP. Albert Handy, an unselfish supporter, idea creator, inspiring me to build the most compassionate, life changing, unbiased, impactful donor-led charity platform ever funded, designed and implemented. Fergus Cloughley and Paul Wallis: true partners and friends and inventors of data flow science. Dan Love, pastor, nurturing my faith in God and compassion for community. Robert Goff, storyteller and teacher. Matt Maloney. Bill York, visionary, networking communities for wellness. Judah Freed, our sagacious editor. Researchers Francis Wong, Ray Kluender, Wes Yin, and Neale Mahoney for rigorous, evidence-based insights.

Judah Freed: I thank all three authors; Allison Sesso and the RIP team; best friend Melissa Mojo; all physicians and healers helping me survive cancer and other ills (covered by Medicare and my Medigap plan). Thanks to RIP, I know how to avoid medical debt.

And we all thank *you* for actually reading acknowledgments!

END
MEDICAL
DEBT

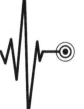

An institution or reform movement that is not selfish, must originate in the recognition of some evil that is adding to the sum of human suffering, or diminishing the sum of happiness.

— CLARA BARTON

INTRODUCTION

Medical Debt:
A Uniquely American Injustice

Allison Sesso
Executive Director, RIP Medical Debt

I felt drawn to the mission of RIP Medical Debt from the first moment I learned about this brilliant and unique approach to addressing unpayable debt from medical bills in America.

Having spent much of my career representing social service providers in New York City, I came to this debt relief work with a deep understanding of the connection between social interventions and health outcomes. I'd evolved a profound appreciation for the growing imbalance between U.S. spending on medical care compared to social programs. I understood that too many people faced severe economic hurdles while measures of health and well-being were going in the wrong direction.

I could not pass up the opportunity to lead an organization with such a dynamic and critical mission. Of course, I could not have known that a weeks after taking the job in January of 2020, the world as we knew it would change from Covid-19.

This pandemic brought the mission of RIP Medical Debt into focus. Covid-19 exacerbated the economic challenges faced by so many. All the Covid layoffs demonstrated the vulnerability of our employer-sponsored health insurance system. Covid tested the healthcare system's ability to respond to a massive medical care crisis. It further exposed health equity issues.

With the fault lines of our modern healthcare system openly exposed, the authors of *End Medical Debt* felt a new edition made good sense. As the new Executive Director of RIP Medical Debt, I knew an update could not be more important in this moment. I could see how the book highlights our mission to end medical debt and to be:

- A source of justice in an unjust healthcare finance system.
- A unique solution for patient-centered healthcare providers.
- A moral force for systemic change.

Medical debt is a uniquely American injustice. It has become an embarrassing feature of our healthcare financing system that forces too many people to endure financial ruin when attempting to meet their health care needs. Our work to obtain and cancel debt not only helps provide economic relief, but it reduces the inevitable avoidance of medical care due to costs, and it removes the substantial mental anguish associated with debt.

People may feel ashamed of having debt because it's generally portrayed as a personal failing. It's not. *Medical debt is a system failure.* This book shows how the system is to blame. That's why RIP now seldom refers to our work as debt "forgiveness," which for some implies wrongdoing. Instead, we're adopting alternative words like relief, cancel, eradicate, and abolish.

We view our work as evolving. Along with providing direct debt relief to people in hardship, we're contributing to the larger conversation around the causes of medical debt.

In *End Medical Debt*, RIP's founders explore the numerous contributing factors to the creation of medical debt — the cost of care, insurance affordability, quality of care, impacts of Covid, employer-based insurance, lack of public understanding, politics, and the structure of the healthcare finance system itself. All of this adds to the problem. The question is, how to fix it?

Few today see our system as working well, but we do not have consensus on what to do about it. How we finance our health care delivery system in America has become immensely complicated. Every bit of progress comes with compromises that undermine enduring success. The Affordable Care Act is a telling example. Misinformation, misunderstanding and growing distrust have undermined our ability to solve this issue in America.

This book does not offer "The Solution" for all the issues of medical debt, but it offers expert perspectives on key contributing factors. The authors lay the groundwork for understanding the main actors in our health system and the incentives driving them — a necessary first step in developing viable solutions.

Thank you, Craig, Jerry and Robert, for taking early risks to get RIP Medical Debt off the ground. Thank you to the Board of Directors for volunteering your time, energy and resources to our growth and entrusting me with execution of this critical mission. Thank you to the incredible team at RIP for showing up every day with passion and impeccable talent. Thank you to all the hospitals partnering with us to provide debt relief to their patients. Thank you to the vast network of partners that support us and cheer us on in so many ways. Most of all, thank you to our donors for your compassion and generosity. We will continue to buy and abolish medical debt for as many people as possible, for as long as this problem exists, while simultaneously doing everything we can to eliminate the need for our work.

— Allison Sesso

*

Creditors have better memories than debtors.

— Benjamin Franklin

PART I

Understanding Medical Debt

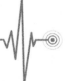

*Debt, n. An ingenious substitute
for the chain and whip of the slavedriver.*

— AMBROSE BIERCE

CHAPTER 1

Seeing Through the Tears

Jerry Ashton

The jaws of medical debt are at America's financial throat. It's as simple and as horrifying as that.

The world of healthcare delivery and economics was turned upside down by Covid-19. What has not changed is that neither job-based insurance nor the Affordable Care Act ("Obamacare") has been up to the task of providing Americans with affordable and accessible healthcare.

I see Covid-19 and the ensuing variants as gas being poured on an existing fire. The pandemic did provide society with one painful benefit, though. It focused unwelcome but needed light on the state of healthcare here in America — how it's dispersed, parceled out, and remains inaccessible for too many.

The first hope for someone falling ill from Covid — or any aliment or injury — is their health insurance. In the USA, health insurance mostly is secured through employment. Most of the 10 million people who lost jobs to Covid in 2020 lost their coverage. FAIR Health says that Covid patients with no insurance ended up with an average of $73,000 in medical debt.

The awareness of healthcare's roadkill — people drowning in unpaid and unpayable medical bills — has moved to the front page. Previously untouched Americans have learned that it's no longer *their* problem (Oh, those poor people). It's *our* problem.

I attribute the stunning mountain of debt, even before Covid, to the for-profit medical model of healthcare delivery — and the politics enabling it. The healthcare industry also is suffering from Covid, but in a very different way. The industry has maxed out its capacity to extract record profits while keeping their "bad debt" losses to an acceptable minimum. They swallow these losses so as not to awaken, or over-alarm, the healthcare consumer.

In the first edition of *End Medical Debt*, we three authors did our best to alert Americans to the unsustainable nature of uncontrolled medical costs, and the tragic amount of debt created by this system. We sought to raise national consciousness. We also described our debt forgiveness charity, RIP Medical Debt.

Our second revised edition first seeks to expand public understanding of the root causes for medical debt. We then weigh the proposed solutions, what could become new U.S. law.

Distracting disinformation abounds, so we ask you to focus on reliable facts over "fake news." We provide verified evidence from authorities we trust. We share insights from people with wisdom that only real-world experience provides. We are more interested in the doers than the talkers.

We hope to affect financial and social practices that cost a loss for every gain we've enjoyed in recent decades. We seek to help America recover from this pandemic as a better people, a better country, a nation without medical debt.

I see no point in creating a "new normal" that reinstates the old normal. The old normal produced our healthcare crisis and brought us consumers to our knees. Let's rethink things.

Our editor describes us three authors as a perfect combination of progressive, conservative and moderate viewpoints. (We have used stronger language referring to one another.) Our differences, he assures me, ensures this book gives you a varied landscape to consider.

In our 12 separate chapters, Craig Antico, Robert E. Goff and I argue our views with supporting evidence. We mostly agree on the causes of medical debt. We agree on debt forgiveness. We differ on solutions, as may you.

Where we all agree is that as America recovers from the pandemic, the crisis in our health care delivery and financing requires us to honestly explore all avenues of thought. We authors do our best to test assumptions about what's right or wrong. We spot common misconceptions. That's not a bad thing. As Leonard Cohen sang, "Everything has a crack in it. That's how the light gets in." We invite you to be brave and honest enough to challenge your ow assumptions on healthcare.

> As America recovers from the pandemic, the crisis in health care delivery and financing requires us to honestly explore all avenues of thought.

We authors offer differing ideas for changing how we deliver and pay for medical services. You may disagree, so let us reason together. We support conversations about a future where medical debt has become an aberration, an oxymoron, rather than today's almost medieval horror show.

How can we possibly let our country do such terrible things to people's health and economic wellbeing? When will come the day we see more "enlightened self-interest" in healthcare?

Doctors agree to a prime directive, "First, do no harm." This oath may inform our work in creating a viable healthcare system. We welcome you to join us in figuring out ways of practicing and financing healthcare that actually will end medical debt.

Painful Truths

Here's where the tears begin. One of the most difficult jobs at RIP is reading the pleas for debt relief. Emails and letters pour in from people across our nation who beg us to help relieve them of their medical debt burdens. Here's a sampling:

- *"My son with MS was discharged with $30,000 in medical bills. He now has no credit, can have no property in his name, has been hounded and pursued by creditors for over three years, and still makes only $12 per hour. This has been a nightmare for all of us, but for a grown man with pride, it's impossible."*

- *"Since my mom's two strokes, we have piled up bill after bill. My dad is the only one paying these bills, and we've lost our house from not paying the mortgage. We now live in an apartment. It's difficult for him to pay medical bills and pay rent."*

- *"The amount owed is about $1,000. If some or all of it were paid, it would be a tremendous burden off my shoulders. I would have my life back. I could rest. All this debt causes me tremendous stress and hopelessness. It's the last thing I think of when I go to bed and the first thing I think of when I wake up."*

- *"I became ill four months before being eligible for Medicare benefits and had no medical coverage at the time. The debts from this illness are overwhelming, and I doubt I will pay them in my lifetime. The surgeon's bill is now in collections, so I cannot go for follow-up tests. There are still bills from two emergency rooms, a seven day hospital stay with various doctors and radiology. All the debts make it impossible for me to meet my obligations. I am now considering bankruptcy."*

One would need a heart of stone not to be reduced to tears by their stories and sense the full desperation in their souls. These are not people in some poor, impoverished country in a land far away. They people are all around us. They are our neighbors, our friends and relatives. They may be us. Millions of Americans are overwhelmed by the cruelty of a healthcare system that until now has resisted every attempt to be corrected, tamed or excised.

Unfortunately, RIP is unable to answer urgent pleas for individual help because we can only cancel older unpaid debt in large batches (or "portfolios"), bought on the secondary debt market for pennies on the dollar. RIP also acquires bad debt directly from healthcare providers. The best we can do for specific individuals is a random hope their old medical bill by chance lands in a portfolio RIP acquires.

Since the Covid pandemic began, the letters and emails RIP receives have not changed in tone or need, nor abated. The Covid tsunami increased the intensity and destruction of medical debt in America. As of publication, RIP has forgiven $5 billion in debt,

> # Millions of Americans are overwhelmed by the cruelty of a healthcare system that until now has resisted every attempt to be corrected or tamed.

helping millions of people, but we can barely scratch the surface. To fix a system we all know is broken, something needs to change, perhaps everything, and it cannot happen soon enough.

Medical Debt Gaining Attention

Lack of health insurance coverage and the costs of care have dominated America's conversation, but unpaid and unpayable medical debt has been little more than a footnote. That people were driven into bankruptcy and even poverty rarely made it into mainstream discussions. The statistics were deemed unfortunate, but not seen as an indictment of the *status quo*. Seems to me all these casualties were accepted as unfortunate collateral damage of "the best healthcare system in the world." We lived with it.

The Covid tsunami increased the intensity and destruction of medical debt.

Then along came Covid. The wail of pandemic deaths caught everybody's attention. Covid's impact on the personal finances of the newly afflicted and newly unemployed became hot breaking headline news, crowding the airways and social media. With this came the realization: *If I lose my job, I'll, lose my insurance!* Then came illness and the thought: *The insurance I have isn't covering my Covid medical costs! Where did this surprise bill come from? The government said it would all be free!*

None of this surprised us at RIP. What was new, however, was a chance to sound the medical debt alarm far more loudly. Executive Director Allison Sesso and the executive team created the "Helping Covid Heroes" campaign. Assisted by data partners, we searched for older debt owed by frontline people in essential jobs. Campaign donors helped RIP cancel about 167,000 medical billing accounts for more than 111,000 individuals in hardship — abolishing medical debt with a face value of $188 million.

Untouched were the billions of unpayable Covid hospital bills that won't come on the secondary debt market for a year or two. I don't know what will be the final tally for Covid-related medical debt. The pandemic is resurging with Delta as I write.

I can guarantee the total will be astounding and an everyday hot topic. This will grow into a white heat as people and society suffer all the costs of unpayable healthcare bills, engendered from Covid within "the best healthcare system in the world."

Medical Debt Counts

Whether one likes or hates the Affordable Care Act, whether one favors or opposes health insurance being reliant on having an employer, concerned people across the political spectrum agree something must be done, now. We are in crisis.

For clear thinking, start with seven evidence-based realities, not biased opinions, about how healthcare is being administered to individuals, families, communities and society at large.

NationalBankruptcy.com in 2019 reported:

1. The United States spends more per capita (per person) on health care than any other country on earth.

2. About 1 in 10 adults delay medical care because of costs.

3. An unexpected $400 to $500 medical bill is too much for too many people to pay, let alone pay in a timely manner.

4. One in five (20 percent) of all working-age Americans with health insurance has trouble paying their medical bills.

5. More than 60 percent of insured Americans with medical bills will deplete most or all of their savings to pay these bills.

6. About 60 percent of people with problems paying medical bills were contacted by a collection agency in the past year.

7. Health insurance annually has become less affordable since 2014, when the Affordable Care Act went into effect.

Out of 255 million adults in the USA in 2019 (U.S. Census), 43 million or 17 percent had near $75 billion in past-due medical debt on their credit reports. CNBC reported on 2019 findings by CompareCards that 33 percent of credit card debt is for medical bills. Sixty percent of these cardholders "had no other way to pay."

> The New York Times reported in 2021 that Americans currently owe $140 billion in medical debt.

Millions of Americans daily must choose between paying health bills or their basic needs like food and shelter. Too many of us don't go to a doctor when ill to avoid the costs, and when they do go, delayed care ends up costing more.

In 2019, RIP estimated the total reported and unreported medical debt accumulated in America over a decade at $1 trillion. Covid has increased this amount by leaps and bounds. *The New York Times* reported in July 2021 that adult Americans currently owe $140 billion in medical debt.

How could all of this happen in one of the world's strongest economies? Follow the money. Our economy values profits and rewards the industries providing them, regardless of social costs. The "common good" is not a consideration when money can be made by those whose only goal is maximizing shareholder value. As I see it, whether or not we hold equity shares, each one of us in America is a stakeholder in the healthcare system.

It doesn't matter if you are a friend or a foe of "capitalism," the *ism* driving our economy. Through money and influence, capitalism created the laws and popular myths that enable and sustain it. Capitalism is so ingrained into our healthcare delivery system that when Covid slammed the economy, inflicting a 4.8 percent GDP drop in the first quarter 2020, *Becker's Healthcare* attributed almost half of that drop to the healthcare sector.

A capitalist may take solace that we have not succumbed to socialism. Bleak satisfaction. Setting aside matters of injustice, advocates of our profit-driven healthcare system are hard pressed to answer a simple question: When Covid struck worldwide, how many people in other industrial nations lost their health insurance when they lost their jobs and had to face frightening medical bills, followed by collection calls? How many? None.

In the first five weeks of Covid lockdowns, 26 million jobs were lost. Because more than half the health insurance purchased in America is through employers, 13 million people suddenly lost their health benefits. That's on top of the 20 million people within our country already without any health insurance.

We pride ourselves in not burdening citizens with high taxes for public health services, as do all other advanced nations, like in Western Europe. Predictably, the dollars "saved" are siphoned off by insurance premiums, high deductibles co-pays, out-of-pocket care expenses, and self-pay balances due after insurance policies provide inadequate coverage. *Whether we pay for our health care through taxes or not, we end up paying the costs.*

Up and down this "chain of pain," as I call it, everyone profits from medical care, especially my own former industry — debt buyers and the debt collection agencies. Someone else's uncollected debt is their potential profit margin. As for the insurance industry, hospital industry, pharmaceutical industry, medical

> As for the insurance industry, hospital industry, pharmaceutical industry, medical supplies and technologies industries, plus Wall Street, do you expect any of them to give up the fat cash cow called the U.S. healthcare system? Not without a fight.

supplies and technologies industries, plus Wall Street, do you expect any of them to give that up the fat cash cow called the U.S. healthcare system? Not without a fight.

A for-profit system may not be so bad if we are getting our money's worth. Are we ?

No, we are not.

In the September 2018 issue of *Managed Care,* Joseph Burns challenged Americans by asking, "Hey, big spender! Why does your quality lag so far behind other countries?" The USA in 2016 spent $10,348 per capita (per person) on medical care, he reports. almost double the per capita average of $5,198 from 11 comparable industrial nations. Citing statistics these countries do better than the USA in crucial health categories, he asked, how do we solve our gap in care?

Adding injury to insult, the citizens in nations with universal healthcare live years longer than Americans. Economics professor John Komlos wrote in a 2015 *PBS NewsHour* column that the average life expectancy in the USA was 79.3 years. In Canada it was 82.2 years. Babies born in Canada on average live three years longer than babies born south of the 49th parallel. Covid has since warped mortality rates.

What label would you put on a healthcare system delivering a better product? Any label you call to mind likely carries baggage. Stop being ruled by corporate misinformation and PR spin. Look instead at the hard evidence of high costs and inefficiencies in the U.S. healthcare system. Look at all the wreckage it leaves behind. Start searching for fresh solutions.

If we don't do this self-examination, if our country returns to the "old normal" as Covid recedes, the loss of this opportunity for change may be worth grieving as much as the loss of life.

The Five Stage of Healthcare Grief

Facing realities in our healthcare system, glaringly exposed by Covid, is like facing the five stages of grief as identified by Dr. Elisabeth Kubler-Ross — *denial, anger, bargaining, depression, acceptance.* The comparison may contain lessons for us.

' The famous Kubler-Ross research dealt with sanely grieving the death of a loved one. When confronted by vast medical debt, shall we not sanely grieve for the loss of the glorious American healthcare system we've cherished for so long?

Can we not legitimately grieve to find our nation among the world's healthcare have-nots? The USA is alone among 33 highly developed countries in not having universal healthcare. Instead, we rank among poor nations like Afghanistan, Cambodia, Chad, Haiti, Iraq, and Zimbabwe. Is this not worth grieving?

Let's explore the structure of the Kubler-Ross five stages of grief to look for any wisdom to be found, any solutions that may be applied to our loss of faith in U.S. healthcare.

• *Denial:* Think beyond trite plays on a river word — da Nile. Ever heard shocking news that you must be taken to a hospital? Ever looked at a hospital bill and said, "This can't be true!" Ever had a care claim denied? Ever had a claim denied for Covid?

"Denial helps us pace our feelings of grief," says Grief.com, "There is a grace in denial. It is nature's way of letting in only as much as we can handle." Denial is the first natural step in beginning the healing process.

Some deny the brokenness of our current system, or they deny the value of universal healthcare. Some defend their belief that our profit-centered system yields the best health care in the world. Or if U.S. care isn't the best, at least we don't have to wait in line to get it. Others deny the contrary evidence to defend their politics or paychecks. Refuting our denials, The Commonwealth Fund says our healthcare system rates as "worst" among 11 high-income nations. Deny that.

The USA is alone among 33 highly developed countries in not having universal healthcare.

Newsweek in 2017 ranked the U.S. system last or near last in access, administrative efficiency, equity, care outcomes, and "especially poor in equality of coverage." The report said 44 percent of low-income Americans have trouble gaining access to coverage, as compared to 26 percent of high-income Americans. Contrast us to UK numbers of seven percent for low income and four percent for high income. Overall, *Newsweek* said the United Kingdom's established National Health Service is the best healthcare system in the world.

Before any workable change can come about in America, we must come to grips with our loss of faith in a healthcare delivery system that's not as great as we want to believe. This might be like the grief of a person coming out of a coma and confronting the bills. We may deny evidence of the total amount now due, but we must pay the price for our care.

> We must come to grips with our loss of faith in a healthcare system that's not as great as we want to believe.

• *Anger*: The shift into anger was exemplified in 2017 by late-night TV host Jimmy Kimmel as Republicans in Congress tried to undo the ACA,.Kimmel pilloried Rep. Bill Cassidy (R-LA), who'd vowed to replace Obamacare with a law that can pass the "Jimmy Kimmel Test."

Kimmel told a live audience, "I don't know what happened to Bill Cassidy... He said he wants coverage for all, no discrimination based on preexisting conditions, lower premiums for middle-class families, and no lifetime caps." He paused. "Guess what? The new [GOP] bill does none of these things."

Republican town halls nationwide had erupted in voter cries for "Repeal and Replace," but the ACA replacement bill did not pass, thanks to one thumbs-down "no" vote by the late Sen. John McCain. His departing good deed will be long remembered.

Psychologist Jeremy Dean suggests an upside to anger may be gaining attention, raising awareness. If so, we need to harness our anger constructively. In our urgent debate over healthcare as we recover from a pandemic, we need more light, not mere heat.

• *Bargaining:* "Please, dear God, please take away the doctor bills, and I promise to ____. If you will rescue me from my wages being garnished, I will ___." (Fill in the blank.) You get the point. In the case of healthcare, is this better than trying to bargain with the devil? For those with the legal power to collect a bill, bargaining a practiced and successful way to extract compliance.

> Republicans gambled on repealing the Affordable Care Act's individual mandate, requiring all Americans to have health insurance. They lost the bet.

In 2017, Republicans gambled on repealing the Affordable Care Act's individual mandate, requiring all Americans to have health insurance. Their trifecta would lower the cost of government, undermine a central pillar of hated Obamacare and finance permanent cuts in corporate tax rates. They lost the bet.

A *Washington Post* opinion piece by University of Michigan law professor Nicholas Bagley questioned the value of 13 million Americans losing their health insurance if the mandate was struck down. Bagley then asked bluntly, "Is the country really better off if millions of people forgo medical care, and millions more go bankrupt, so corporations can pay lower taxes? ...Those are the stakes of the game."

The GOP lawsuits against the individual mandate ultimately failed in June 2021 when the U.S. Supreme Court for the third time ruled the ACA mandate to have insurance *is* constitutional.

Republicans in congress threatened a government shutdown in 2018 by using the Children's Health Insurance Program (CHIP) as a bargaining chip. CHIP offers low-cost insurance for children in families earning too much for Medicaid, but too little to afford private insurance. In some states, CHIP covers pregnant women. The GOP did not bargain on public support for children.

I believe it's time to stop using health for political bargaining. History has taught us that however well things turn out for the principals in such bargains, the general public loses.

I admit to stretching the Kubler-Ross model, for such political maneuvering is not bargaining — it's hostage-taking. Bargaining involves offering something valuable or precious in return.

• *Depression:* The simplest definition of depression is when people fall into an unhappy, hopeless mental state. As Grief.com says, "Empty feelings present themselves, and grief enters into our lives... deeper than we ever imagined." Depression from grief may feel endless, feel like forever, but it's not a "mental illness." It's a healthy response to a genuine loss.

We at RIP feel the depression and hopelessness out there. We read emailed cries for help from people who discover us, find out what we do and pray for us to help them:

• *"I had a heart attack and two cardiac procedures in the last year. My husband had a heart attack two years before."*

• *"I've had cancer for three years. The bills are in collections."*

• *"I'm on a fixed income. I struggle to pay the past-due bills."*

• *"I have no money to my name. I fear becoming homeless."*

America has suffered economic depressions and recessions, most recently from Covid shutdowns. I can't fathom the amount of pain and misery we may go through as individuals, families and as a society before we reach a semblance of recovery. I feel depressed by even writing about it.

• *Acceptance*: Only when we go through the next and final stage of grief, acceptance of facts, will we ever turn things around. How can we change reality if we don't accept it's real?

For some, "acceptance" implies a passive surrender to some unthinkable possibility. For others, it means giving permission for hostile forces to have their way with us. For other, acceptance is the frightening realization we no longer have any choice.

> An essential building block for a better American society will be a medical system recognizing healthcare is a human right.

I ascribe to Reinhold Niebuhr's poem, as adapted into the Serenity Prayer. "God, grant me the serenity to accept the things I cannot change, the courage to change the things I can, and the wisdom to know the difference."

In the case of our healthcare system, acceptance for me means coming to terms with the truth of our situation. That's not surrender. It's engaging with the reality I wish didn't exist. Let's admit hard facts and move on.

I accept that anger and rage draw attention to our grievances, but furious feelings change little or nothing if our energy is never put to good use through positive action. I accept that bargaining with the current system has not produced a satisfying resolution, further feeding our grievances. I also accept that feeling depressed and victimized about our dire plight is normal, but that can be an emotional trap.

Let us agree to face all the facts as best as we can, understand them, and accept the things beyond our reach to change, *yet*.

The next step, individually and collectively, will be to dig in deep and find the courage to change those things we can change — inch by inch, brick by brick, day by day.

I believe an essential building block for a better American society will be a medical system recognizing healthcare is a basic human right. I believe no one should exhaust their life savings on medical bills, not as millions of Americans do annually. I believe no person should lose their home, go bankrupt or suffer material or personal losses because they had the misfortune of contracting an illness or getting injured. The only tears I want in future are tears of joy when such burdens are gone and forgotten.

You may not agree with my solution of national healthcare. You may prefer instead the solutions from my co-authors, or you may have even better ideas. The starting place is acceptance that our existing healthcare system is in crisis, and action is urgently needed to end the crippling hardship of medical debt.

Praying to know the difference between what is possible and impossible, asking for strength of purpose to inspire political will, I invite us to change what we can. We can find serenity in knowing that ending medical debt is not America's first moon shot.

We can do this.

What can be added to the happiness
of a man [sic] who is in health, out of debt,
and has a clear conscience?

— ADAM SMITH

CHAPTER 2

Medical Debt is the Enemy of Everyone

Robert E. Goff

M edical debt is the mortal enemy of the patient, the physician, the hospital, the community, the state, and the nation.

When we think about others' debts, we tend to say the debts are their personal responsibility. If they're unable to pay the debt, it's their problem. (We make it a *You* problem, not a *Me* problem.)

Society tells us a problem with personal debt is a direct result of bad decisions, poor personal financial habits, profligate spending, living beyond one's means, or compulsive debting. We blame those with medical debt for their bad choice of buying substandard health insurance, or else for not purchasing any health insurance at all.

We say the consequences of debt are rightly visited on the debtor. Whatever the impact — canceled credit cards, low credit, wage garnishment — it's all on them. Personal responsibility.

Is this true? In the big picture, we individuals and society both bear the costs and burdens of personal "bad debt." For individuals who fall into arrears in their payments, who just cannot pay their financial obligations, unpaid debt means their ability to buy goods and services is curtailed or perhaps ended. If new credit is not extended, the person must live on cash.

> When Covid-19 disproportionally impacted lower social-economic brackets (initially people of color and the elderly), more patients than usual who needed care lacked adequate health benefits coverage.

For any business, any debt that's not paid by the customer creating it becomes a cost to the enterprise extending credit. The business recoups its loss by raising prices on products or services for all future customers. The business may stop its loss by not providing goods or services to a debtor, disciplining patrons not paying their bills. In such cases, the consequences of unpaid bills fall on the debtor and creditor, usually ending there.

This just does not apply to medical care services. Personal debt from being unable to pay for necessary healthcare services is the cause of medical debt. It is *not* a voluntary debt.

The range of consequences from all unpayable medical bills extends far beyond individuals and service providers. Medical debt ripples outward, adversely affecting physicians, hospitals, communities, potentially requiring intervention by government, and that impacts us taxpayers.

Covid brought into full clarity the consequences of desperately needing medical care without an adequate ability to pay.

Medical providers during the pandemic, as expected, provided care regardless of a patient's ability to pay. When Covid-19 disproportionally impacted the lower social-economic brackets (initially people of color and the elderly), more patients than usual who needed care lacked adequate health benefits coverage.

Covid patients on Medicaid and Medicare have been covered by government programs. Covid patients with commercial insurance, including plans bought through the ACA Marketplace, have been expected to rely on their private coverage, exposing them to their plans' deficiencies, such as high deductibles.

Other Covid patients have been caught in confusion over their eligibility for charity care, problems from sloppy billing, and even outright exploitation — resulting in patients being left financially exposed for their Covid-related care. Those most at risk include the "long haul" Covid patients having to pay out-of-pocket for care after their hospital discharge.

Covid vaccinations can incur medical debt, too. *The New York Times* in December 2020 reported "surprise bills" were happening. Some care providers receiving basic federal coverage for the costs of vaccinations found ways to sweeten the pot. Some added a "facility fee" if the administering physician was a hospital employee. They added an "Emergency Room fee" if that's where the injections were given. These fees were not covered by the federal guidelines, or by commercial insurance, so financial exposure landed on the patient. I believe this practice has not yet been curtailed for Delta.

The Debt Daisy Chain

Medical debt is not like a debt incurred by buying a big screen TV one cannot afford. It should not be treated the same way.

Medical debt largely results from unplanned, involuntary events, often an illness or accident. It is *not* a choice. Illness is never chosen.

Sure, certain lifestyle choices, personal habits and emotional habits can lessen the chances of ill health. Smoking, drinking, illicit drugs, unhealthy foods, and all other risky behaviors are private choices. However, no one consciously volunteers to be ill. No one volunteers for a costly personal injury accident. Medical debt is not about living beyond one's means. Medical debt is about staying alive.

If people are unable to accept personal financial responsibility for the economic results of medical efforts to restore (or try to restore) them back to good health, medical debt is incurred.

Covid brought into clarity the consequences of desperately needing medical care without an adequate ability to pay, which causes medical debt.

• *Having medical debt deters access to medical services.* Owing medical debt, patients often wait until a condition becomes acute, when the care of last resort is the emergency room. The ER is the most costly, least appropriate for non-urgent care. More debt.

Unlike private sellers of goods or services, medical providers do not cut off a debtor from all care. Medical debt may affect when and where a debtor receives care, but medical services are still available in some form. Physicians cannot ethically let us suffer. Hospitals by law must treat all who enter the emergency room.

Among all medical care providers, physicians and hospitals bear the heaviest economic burden from medical debt. Their patients' unpaid bills then impact the rest of the healthcare system.

Unlike commercial ventures, hospitals and physicians do not routinely recover losses by increasing prices for the patients who can pay their bills. The cost sharing does not end there.

In today's system of private and government health insurance, care payments are set by contracts or regulations. Medicare and Medicaid reimbursements to medical providers use formulas tied to their costs for delivering care. Insurance plans pay the lowest rates possible, based on set competitive financial factors. Care providers cannot simply raise their fees to cover accumulating losses.

For individuals, medical debt is a barrier to good health. Poor health means a loss of job productivity, maybe less or no income, reducing contributions to family wellbeing, reducing contributions to the economics of society through employment taxes.

For hospitals, unpaid costs for care reduce their fiscal viability. Some seek taxpayer support through government programs to stay viable. Taxpayer support translates into higher taxes. Businesses avoid expanding or relocating in areas with high local taxes, which reduces desirability for economic development. A high proportion of medical indigents in a community reduces its allure to physicians. Less community health care cuts its desirability for workers and for business. Fewer jobs depress the local economy, further weakening the ability of residents to pay for insurance and medical care.

Consider the interconnected social and economic daisy chain of medical debt in America. What impacts one impacts all.

Gaps in Medical Care

When medical insurance is lacking, or has gaps in coverage that limit protection against financial hardships, the economics weigh heavily on a person's decision whether or not to seek medical care. If care is sought, insurance coverage, or its lack, affects the decision to follow treatment plans or fill prescriptions.

Gaps in health insurance, including high deductibles, coupled with the increasingly byzantine rules for full insurance coverage, impact those struggling with their health decisions. One in three Americans postpone seeking medical care for themselves or family members due to the high cost of medical care, according to a 2014 Gallup poll reported in *The Daily Caller*. That percentage has risen since enactment of the Affordable Care Act (ACA). Increasing delays in treatment are generally attributed to higher ACA insurance deductibles. Higher insurance deductibles increase medical debt. Deductibles, regardless of amount, are a patient's personal financial responsibility.

Higher insurance deductibles increase medical debt.

Failures to follow recommended treatments, like not taking prescriptions, are not solely due to costs, but cost are a large part of the reason for non compliance. A 2015 National Center for Health Statistics study found eight percent of Americans don't take their medicines as prescribed because they can't afford them. Nearly 20 percent of all prescriptions never get filled. Poor self-care leads to poor health.

Delayed or missed care raises costs by raising illness severity, which contributed to higher than expected non-Covid deaths at the pandemic's height. When delayed care at last is sought, the costs are inevitably higher, the outcomes predictably poorer. More extensive and expensive care increases medical debt for everyone.

The poor or near-poor are not the only ones delaying care due to its high cost. Gallup reported that in 2014, the first full year of the Affordable Care Act ("Obamacare"), among middle-class people earning between $30,000 and $75,000, 38 percent delayed care due to costs, up from 33 percent in 2013. Among those earning above

$75,000 annually, about 28 percent told Gallup they delayed care, much more than the 17 percent in 2013. So, roughly a third of all "affluent" Americans delay care due to costs, regardless of the effects on themselves or society.

Economic impacts continue once treatment starts. The Cancer Support Center found 20 percent of cancer patients skipped advised treatments, fearing out-of-pocket costs. Almost 50 percent said their costs were more than expected. Cost concerns delayed screening tests, which delayed treatment, reducing treatment effectiveness. In cancer care, early detection and treatment yields the best outcomes. Fear of medical debt caused later disease discovery, later treatment, and less favorable outcomes. Gaps in care are deadly.

An American Cancer Society study released in 2019 reported medical financial hardships impact more than 100 million people from increased stress or delaying care because of costs.

Covid adds another dimension to insured patients' risk of fiscal hits and setback in their physical wellbeing. The Centers for Disease control in September reported that by June 2020, concerns about Covid-19 led about 41 percent of U.S. adults to delay or to avoid medical care, including urgent or emergency care, contributing to an additional 10 percent increase in deaths. Covid patients get economically slammed. A Covid hospitalization too often is a gateway to medical debt. Any deficiency in health insurance coverage can soon swallow up an individual and family's financial resources.

Medical debt could even deny you a Covid vaccination. In 2021, Boulder Medical Center in Colorado cancelled a vaccination for Michael Rogan, a 72 year-old cancer patient, due to an outstanding $243 bill. When the news went public, the hospital apologized and vaccinated him, said *Becker's Hospital CFO Report*. That's good for him. How many other hospitals have held vaccinations hostage to clear unpaid balances? How many died due to unpaid bills?

Covid-19's Triple Whammy

Covid hit medical care providers with a triple whammy.

First, as hospital's stand-by capacity went for Covid patients, lately for Delta, elective procedures were eliminated or curtailed for safety. Cautious patients deferred planned procedures. Profitable patient volume fell or did not materialize.

Second, as stressed providers competed for limited supplies of personal protective equipment (PPE) like masks and gowns, plus scarce supplies like oxygen, costs soared. Price gouging and counterfeits, like fake N95 masks, became common news stories.

The third whammy adding financial pressure to hospitals and physicians was the higher level of bad debt from the Covid patients unable to pay their bills, often from job loss. The economy had improved by the 2021 Delta variant surge, yet all this bad debt adds to the care costs daisy chain. Covid points out the fallacy that today's system of hospital financing matches the medical needs of our communities. That is not true.

Where waves of Covid ravaged communities, non-emergency care mostly stopped to leave medical capacity available for potential and real Covid cases. The shift eliminated usual hospital revenue from other procedures and non-Covid patients. Where the spike in cases was not extreme, hospitals had empty beds and empty procedure

> Covid points out the fallacy that today's system of hospital financing matches the medical needs of communities. That is not true.

34

rooms, resulting in empty bank accounts. No patients, no revenue, but hospitals still had the expenses of standby readiness for a surge, whether it occurred or not.

When Covid hit, hospitals were financially devastated. Their

When Covid hit, hospitals were financially devastated.

median operating margins dropping 55.6 percent in early 2020, reported consultants Kaufman Hall. The fiscal blow on hospitals was cushioned by passage of the CARES Act (Coronavirus Aid Relief and Economic Security), yet median operating margins still dropped 16.6 percent.

As for individuals, medical debt drives calculations of care vs. cost. When medical costs outstrip an individual's and family's economic ability to pay, the resulting medical debt gets between a patient and necessary medical care. "Should I go to the doctor?" becomes "Can I afford to see the doctor?" "Should I fill this prescription?" becomes "Can I afford to fill it?" Too often, cost wins out over care. A Covid cough gets ignored until it's too late.

Consider the human costs in desperate situations. In Boston on July 4, 2018, UPI reported, a woman's leg was caught in between a subway car and the platform, ripping her flesh to the bone. Crying in agony, she pleaded with her rescuers *not* to call an ambulance. "It's $3,000," she cried. "I can't afford that!"

The CARES Act provided for the uninsured. But the people with private insurance who needed Covid care learned the limitations of their benefit plans. Thankfully, some insurers, if temporarily, implemented wavers of deductibles, co-pays, and other coverage limits. Such considerations were far from universal, and these began ending as vaccines became available. For Covid patients, their illness too often was an opportunity for accumulating medical debt.

Medical Debt Poverty Trap

For individuals, the ultimate economic consequence of medical debt could be impoverishment. After personal and family resources are exhausted, if impoverished, they are eligible for publicly funded medical insurance, like Medicaid, or maybe charity assistance.

Medicaid benefits tend to be more complete than commercial health insurance — often without deductibles. However, Medicaid limits the choice of providers. It carries negative social connotations. Still, the coverage is often better than employer-provided insurance. To receive Medicaid, though, you do have to be in poverty.

Comprehensive insurance with high deductibles contributes to delayed care from money worries — increasing illness and depleting financial resources, even to the extent of impoverishment, which is what makes one eligible for Medicaid.

Medicaid or charity assistance is not an escape. Such help comes to the rescue only after the patient or the family has "spent down," depleting their financial reserves, perhaps due to limited or absent insurance coverage. Seems to me bitterly ironic that families must be economically destroyed before they are eligible for the care that would have avoided such harm in the first place. Medical indigence can trap individuals and families into actual poverty.

Medical debt affects the whole economic ecosystem.

The CARES Act refreshingly mitigated financial exposure for the uninsured. Eligibility does not require the same forced impoverishment as Medicaid, a temporary benefit unique to Covid.

The truth is that access to medical charity usually comes only after a patient or family is deemed insolvent or in poverty, too often from medical debt. Most charities do not cover any medical debts accumulated prior to entering their programs. If they do, they only cover medical bills. Higher costs of living caused by illness are not covered, nor is loss of income from caring for a family member.

The involuntary physical burden of an illness or accident stays with individuals and families. The wider economic costs are borne by the entire community and our full nation of taxpayers. Medical debt affects the whole economic ecosystem.

> # Poorer care for poorer people costs all the taxpayers more.

Taxes fund state and federal government healthcare programs. The ACA, *Obamacare*, dramatically increased the number of people eligible for Medicaid on a state-by-state basis, mainly those near the poverty line and below it. Many state legislatures provided hospitals with funds for the indigent. As with Medicaid, state hospital support programs are financed by taxpayers.

When hospitals provide charity care, under current rules, the costs may be offset by higher fees to patients' insurance companies. That offset becomes higher premiums paid by insured people. If a hospital cannot pass on its charity costs, where Medicaid payments are insufficient, government assistance may keep a hospital's doors open as a community resource and major employer.

Public resentment of tax burdens has restrained Medicaid reimbursements. Low Medicaid payments are not attractive to providers, so a fraction of local medical providers participates in the program. Inadequate Medicaid reimbursement means indigent patients often are limited to public or charity clinics, or episodic ER care. They lack a stable physician-patient relationship for the "continuum of care" and preventative care. The lack contributes to medical debt.

Low Medicaid reimbursements in some places attract only care providers with less desirable training or talent, not those able to earn a living with payments from insurance or affluent patients.

Poorer care for poorer people costs all the taxpayers more. The medical gap trap impacts everyone in American society.

Taking Unfair Advantage

Employees paying high payroll deductions for health coverage often enjoy a false sense of security. After the deductible, they think, the insurance will protect their financial wellbeing. Not so. All coverage has "rules" limiting protections. Intended to keep down insurance premiums. The rules may shock workers when reality hits.

Many insurance plans refuse to pay for care, even if medically necessary, if it falls outside their own self-dictated restrictions. Out-of-network care providers may not be covered except in proven life-threatening emergencies, or with specific pre-authorizations.

What parent in Refreshingly middle of the night is going to think it through when a child has profuse bleeding, abdominal pain, or fever spike? They rush to the emergency room, the only provider of medical care outside normal business hours for physicians.

Under health insurance rules, coverage for care in emergencies may not be provided if the insurance company asserts, after the fact, the event did not threaten life or limb. The rule may avert an insurer from accepting fiscal responsibility for paying your medical bill.

Much to our detriment, we seldom invest time to understand the limitations of our health insurance coverage, all the nuances. If a family member or ourselves gets ill or injured, feeling urgency, we may accept care without realizing the financial consequences.

Unethical care providers may exploit our ignorance of plan coverage. They may misrepresent participation in a plan to "capture" patients and related care revenue.

Phrases like "participating" or "will bill insurance" or "will take insurance" may sound reassuring to the patient, but these terms do not guarantee what most patients think.

A patient who receives care may get a nasty and costly shock. If insurance unexpectedly denies a bill, the patient finds a physician or clinic is not covered by their policy. The patient suddenly discovers the bill is their own responsibility.

Patients may find themselves on the short end if a physician cuts a deal to accept whatever insurance pays. That deal may not cover any service providers who are not in-network. The patient gets a surprise bill. *The New York Times* reported on a patient whose surgeon agreed to accept whatever insurance paid, but used an out-of-network assistant surgeon who billed $117,000.

To their credit, the insurance company, Aetna, takes an aggressive stance against enticing patients into financial traps. They filed suit in New York against two doctors, in-network Dr. Ramin Rak and out-of-network Dr. Shuriz Hishmeh. Dr. Rak used Dr. Hishmeh as a co-surgeon on procedures. For instance, Dr. Rak got $183,294 in-network. Dr. Hishmeh got more than $1.1 million out-of-network, said Crain's *New York Business*, reporting that the patient was liable for all out-of-network surgery costs above Aetna's allowable rates.

> We seldom invest the time to understand the limitations of our health insurance coverage. Unethical care providers may exploit our ignorance of plan coverage.

Even where insurance does step up to protect patients by paying the bills, abusing out-of-network billing inevitably results in higher health insurance premiums for everyone.

A 2019 report on PBS *Bill of the Month* gave a relevant example. Alexa Kasdan had a cold and a sore throat. While some medical professionals may say it was not medically necessary, her physician took a throat culture for a rapid strep test, and sent it to a laboratory that was not contracted with her insurance company. The lab sent her a surprise bill for $28,395. Her insurer cut a check for $25,865. Her 10 percent co-pay left her owing a $2,530 balance.

Her doctor's office called her and said not to worry about the balance. The lab had agreed to accept the $25,865 as full payment, and even generously sent a courier to pick up the check. In other words, insurance is paying the tab, so no need to do more.

Financial abuses of out-of-network billing result in higher health insurance premiums for everyone.

Ms. Kasdan did do more. She talked to a public TV reporter. The aired story said her regular in-network laboratory, LabCorp, would have charged $653 for "all the ordered tests, or an equivalent." (From curiosity, I checked a useful price comparison tool at MDSave.com and found a rapid strep test in her locale carried an average cost of $75.)

Ms. Kasdan went public with alleged financial abuse by the laboratory and her physician. Only then did her insurance company, BCBS of Minnesota, announced it would take more interest in how well it was "protecting" the policy holder's premium dollar.

ProPublica in 2020 reported on a Covid test given to a physician at his place of employment, Physicians Premier ER in Austin. As a pathologist, he knew the material cost of the test was about $8. His insurance was billed $10,9894, and it was paid, no questions asked. As a reference, Medicare would pay about $43 for the same test.

Profiting From Covid

Unfortunately, Covid brought out the scammers and exploiters, only some of whom have been exposed. Covid also brought to light the incompetence putting patients at financial risk.

The situation is not black and white. As one example, many insurance companies, to their credit, have waived co-payments and deductibles related to Covid detection and treatment. However, patients may have to fight to get coverage on high hospital charges. Being assertive helps patients avoid medical debt.

This can be complicated. A positive Covid test means the patient will get care and the bills will be covered. Urgent or emergency care provided before a Covid test is done may not be covered. Early in the pandemic, hospitals could not get Covid test materials, so no testing. No test means no waiver of the patient's financial responsibility.

Granted, billing and coding errors for Covid lab work result in claims being denied, like not linking a test to covered medical care. There also are improper practices. *Yahoo News* in 2020 reported on a high school science teacher in New York City, Stephanie Nickolas, who got negative test results from the CityMD, listed by NYC for free Covid tests. A month later, she got a $300 bill, which her insurer had paid. She called CityMD, which said it was a mistake and ignore it. She did not ignore the lab being paid for a "free" Covid test. She blew the whistle. Self-advocacy helps catch incompetence.

Self-serving medical providers can be unscrupulous. *The Texas Tribune* in 2020 reported a patient's doctor visit for a $175 Covid test drew an \$11,000 bill, which the patient's insurance company paid without protest. If that patient had a deductible, by the way, they could have been on the hook upwards to \$2,200 or more.

Collections and Bankruptcy

If people do not pay their medical bills, collections begin!

Aggressively pursued medical debt can destroy the stability and security of individuals and families. Collectors compel debtors to choose between paying the rent, food, transportation, childcare, or other overdue bills. To satisfy collection demands, those with limited means may feel forced to miss a mortgage payment or not put tires on the car. Some give up on even trying to be a "responsible" person, refusing to answer the phone or open the mail.

Bloomberg News in 2014 ran a story on a William Piorun facing an impossible choice between paying for his mortgage or paying for his medications, which cost \$20,000 a month. He had coverage, but his co-pay was more than \$1,000 per month. How can he live?

> Medical debt on a credit report can prevent earning the money to pay off that medical debt.

Urgency rises when collections begin. A professional bill collector has one goal: Collect the monies owed to their client, regardless of consequences from life decisions they force debtors to make.

Adding to the injury, many employers check credit reports on prospective employees before they hire them. Glassdoor reported in 2018 that almost 60 percent of all employers do credit checks on job candidates. They presume that those under financial stress, or showing difficulty with personal finances, may be less responsible or more likely to commit white-collar crime, so they are less desirable. Medical debt on a credit report can prevent earning the money to pay off that medical debt.

Medical debt ultimately gets paid by us taxpayers.

A 2019 report by Lorie Konish on CNBC noted high healthcare bills are the top reason people are taking money out of retirement accounts or else filing bankruptcy. *The Journal of General Internal Medicine* reported 137 million Americans faced hardship in 2019 because of medical costs — nearly 40 percent of all Americans.

Bankruptcy releases debt, but it stays on a credit report 10 years. Credit is denied, negatively affecting reconstruction of their lives. Forget about a mortgage or a car loan, and that's for starters. Even after all the debt is discharged, enduring punishments from personal bankruptcy are anything but an actual "clean slate."

If you think the worse consequence of unpaid medical bills is bankruptcy, a 2017 story in *Miami New Times* reported medical debt in South Florida was the leading cause of homelessness. It beat out mental illness and drug abuse as the top reasons. Medical debt beat out job loss as the primary cause of Miami homelessness.

Personal Responsibility

Personal responsibility matters, yet debt from necessary medical care is innately different than debt from living beyond one's means. Survival not vanity is the real cause of medical debt. Whether or not the economic impacts are noticed, medical debt affects us all. The Covid pandemic further distressed the healthcare system.

Healthcare is an interconnected system. Medical debt drives up insurance premiums and deductibles. Medical debt drives up taxes for Medicare and Medicaid, drives up our taxes for saving local care institutions. Personal medical debt does not stop with the debtor. Medical debt ultimately gets paid by us taxpayers.

All of us pay for medical debt, if not our own, then the medical debt of others. As rising medical costs outstrip individuals' ability to pay, the impacts go beyond the amount of any medical bill. We may argue about the costs of health care. We may argue about solutions. Debate is good but not enough. *Medical debt is the elephant in the room nobody wants to talk about.* We cannot get around it.

Commercial insurance, Medicare, Medicaid, and charity care promise protection and relief from medical impoverishment. But the social safety net has gaping holes for individuals, and communities pay the price, as does our entire nation. Medical debt is the enemy of everyone. That's not what we expect here in America.

CHAPTER 3

Debt Mountains Cause Healthcare Deserts

Craig Antico

We all bear the costs of medical debt, as Robert Goff says. Why, then, do we ignore and allow material hardships from debt to fall heaviest upon certain known groups of people? Doesn't seem to me like we all bear the costs of medical debt fairly. Don't we have a collective responsibility to right this wrong?

Every year, between 15 to 20 percent of all Americans from all walks of life suffer inordinate medical debt that affects their psyche, behavior and wellbeing. This impact is magnified by social determinants like isolation, income insecurity, transportation insecurity, education level, access to healthcare, and living environment — often influenced by gender and racial disparities.

We're finally starting to understand the consequences of severe medical debt in people's lives.

Researchers at the Economics and Public Policy departments of UCLA, UC/Berkeley, University of Chicago, and MIT have released the preliminary finding of an economic impact study that measures the effects of medical debt forgiveness by RIP (see Section II). The findings shed light on how medical debt affects people's wellbeing. I believe these findings should influence public policy.

A major finding is that insurmountable "debt mountains" may undermine our wellbeing. The debt itself may cause us to behave as if we're living in "healthcare deserts." We may choose not to access needed healthcare, even if available in our community, for fear of the costs and stress resulting from more medical debt.

Who is buried on Debt Mountain? People in poverty and with limited public support and resources. Youth in their late twenties. Those with severe diseases (like cancer, mental illness or addiction). Forty million working-class Americans earning an average of $12 an hour with no company-provided health insurance. Veterans denied VA coverage. All these people are buried on debt mountains.

Ailments Atop Debt Mountains

For almost every age, gender, race, and class in the USA, the mountains of medical debt keep growing. People with serious and chronic ailments of body and mind too often end up buried under mountains of debt,

Two examples suggest the scale of the mountain.

• *Cancer:* As you may know, or one close to you may know, a cancer diagnosis is devastating. Next, you start getting and paying the bills. A study in the *Journal of Clinical Oncology* confirmed the bills increase patients' stress and increase early mortality.

At least a third of the cancer patients with insurance pay more out-of-pocket for treatments than they expected to spend. A Duke University survey found that patients were paying an average of 11 percent of their household income on out-of-pocket costs for cancer treatment. The cancer patients reporting the most financial distress were spending 30 percent of their income on health care.

• *Mental Illness and Addiction*: Few health plans cover mental health or addiction treatment services. The few plans that do rarely cover treatment to the full extent deemed medically necessary by consumers, caregivers, and doctors.

Such bills do not show up anywhere in medical debt statistics. Bills are paid by friends and family, or from savings, or credit cards, or selling a house. Mental health care often is out-of-network since most providers want to be paid upfront. If uninsured or underinsured, you or a loved one might not get needed help.

A Kaiser Family Foundation analysis of suicide and intentional injuries found 82 percent have more than $1,000 in out-of-pocket expenses (OOP), and 16 percent have OOP expenses over $5,000. The severe mental health conditions associated with the highest OOP expenses are suicide attempts, psychotic disorders and dementia.

All this cost burden is disconcerting. Nearly a fifth of our total adult population report mental health issues. An insured employee with mental health care spending may have out-of-pocket costs passing $5,000, double that of a physical health issue. Researchers at RIP and Definitive Healthcare calculate that of 35 million inpatient visits to U.S. hospitals, at least 38 percent "present" psychosis as a primary or a secondary diagnosis.

> The study's cancer patients reporting the most financial distress were spending 30% of their income on health care.

Few of us are comfortable discussing how medical debt from mental illness and addiction are debilitating U.S. families.

Debt of Necessity

Medical debt generally fits into a larger category that we call "debt of necessity" — an unexpected expense to meet unexpected emergencies and living expenses. A debt of necessity could include a credit card debt or payday loan for repairing a vehicle, or putting food on the table.

More than 50 percent of our fellow citizens in this country chronically have at least two of the three criteria that RIP uses to determine debt forgiveness:

• *Low earnings.*

• *Zero net worth*

• *High out-of-pocket medical expenses as a percentage of gross income.*

When I consider the people that RIP helps, I wonder how they get by when facing unpayable debts of necessity like medical debt. Turns out, a lot of them don't.

Some 15 million people annually lose their life savings because of medical debt. When it comes to medical bills, thanks to our broken healthcare system, crowdfunding has become the insurance policy of last resort. How often can we appeal to our friends and family to rescue us?

How Much Medical Debt is Owed?

When hospitals and physicians provide care services for which they do not get paid, that's "uncompensated care," and it generally falls into two categories — *charity care* and *bad debt.*

• **Charity care** services, provided free by hospitals, at cost, are paid from an annual budget line for uncompensated charity care in qualified hardship cases. Pre-Covid, this averaged about $25 billion per year, and equaled about 2 percent of all hospital expenses. Kaiser

Health Network reported that nonprofit hospitals in 2019 sent bills for $2.7 billion to patients who likely qualified for free or discounted care, putting these patients at risk of medical debt.

• *Bad debt* is the amount left unpaid for hospital care services. A hospital charge is calculated from the "master price" for a service, minus any discounts, to create a "reasonable and customary" charge. Whatever portion of that charge is not compensated, whether paid by insurance or the patient, becomes bad debt. Hospital bad debt may be submitted for collections, and so unpaid accounts land on credit reports. (An unpaid account does not become bad debt in the same year the bill was generated, but it likely will over time.)

> Only about 60% of all medical bills get paid in a given year.

• *Hospitals.* To help you understand how our hospitals produce medical debt, I want to share a healthcare insider's rule-of-thumb for the annual hospital revenue cycle.

Of the total amount billed as "reasonable and customary" that uninsured (self-pay) patients owe in a given year, about 10 percent of the bills will be paid that year. Of the total amount billed to those with private insurance, after insurance pays its part, less than half of all that balance after insurance (BAI) will be paid that year. Only about 60 percent of all medical bills get paid in a given year.

Applying this rule, given an annual average of $500 billion billed to patients, the 40 percent unpaid balance is $200 billion. It's all the patient's responsibility, and it can become medical debt.

• *Physicians.* The amount people owe physicians is almost equal to hospital bad debt. My co-author Robert E. Goff, long a healthcare administrator, has a rule of thumb on private physician bad debt:

$40,000 per doctor per year. Given about 1 million active physicians in the USA, according to Kaiser Family Foundation. This means $40 billion in physician bad debt every year.

Now add the $200 billion annually in hospital bad debt to $40 billion annually in physician bad debt. We get $240 billion medical debt per year. Multiply by ten years, then subtract the 20 percent for bills likely paid over a decade, you get about $2 trillion in debt.

• *Credit reports.* Another way to calculate the total outstanding medical debt is from the amount in collections, as identified from credit reports. (This excludes credit card charges to pay medical bills and court judgments). I know from years in collections that one in ten medical bills in collections get reported to credit agencies.

The Journal of the American Medical Association (JAMA) in July 2021 published original research that estimated pre-Covid medical debt in 2020 at $140 billion. Four university researchers analyzed a tenth of aggregated medical debt reported to TransUnion from 2009 to 2020. The economic impact study found medical debt was highest in states with the least Medicaid. (*Full disclosure*: This independent academic study happened because the four economics researchers contacted RIP in 2016. Jerry tells the story in Chapter 9.)

Debt never dies. Barring interventions — like debt cancellation by a hospital or physician, or debt forgiveness by RIP — individuals owe medical debt for as long as their psyches allow. The unpaid bills live in file cabinets, on kitchen tables, on their minds.

Uninsured and Underinsured

The Commonwealth Fund reports that 68 million people in our county are underinsured or uninsured.

The Fund considers people "underinsured" if their deductible equals more than five percent of their gross income, which comprise most of the underinsured. Other people are underinsured if their deductible passes 10 percent of their gross income, if they earn more than two times the current Federal Poverty Level (FPL) guidelines (Healthcare.com). Underinsured people get more care bills.

The underinsured with a lot of medical debt include people making poor health care choices from being uninformed about medical services, from not understanding what their health insurance plan covers, and primarily from using services (knowingly and unknowingly) from costly out-of-network care providers.

I can confirm this from all my work at RIP. For every healthcare debt portfolio RIP purchases, each account is scrutinized by analytics

> # The middle class is most likely to have high out-of-network bills, which if long left unpaid will become medical debt.

of consumer credit data and social determinant data to assess who qualifies for debt relief, who gets the golden envelopes.

From this body of evidence, I've drawn some conclusions about who suffers from medical debt, and how it harms them.

• *Middle Class:* Most of the underinsured people are part of the "middle class," which comprises less than half of the U.S. adult population. They earn from 200 percent to 350 percent of the poverty level. Despite a good income, the underinsured spend at least five percent of their gross income on out-of-pocket medical costs.

About 20 to 25 percent of the debt we cancel at RIP is for people in the middle class. They qualify for our debt relief because a large percent of their gross income goes for out-of-pocket expenses and debt service. Wanting the best care, they will "pay" for it, even if the doctor or service is not fully covered under their health plan. That "sensible decision" for better health can be costly. The middle class is most likely to have high out-of-network bills, which if long left unpaid will become medical debt.

• *Working Class:* About 44 million Americans are "working class," and few receive health insurance from their employer. Under the ACA, they may purchase health insurance on their own through a Marketplace portal. Budget policies with high deductibles may leave them underinsured. RIP forgives lots of their medical debt.

• *Youth:* The youngest, healthiest workers in their twenties too often opt-out of health insurance, or they pick the lowest-premium plan with the highest deductibles. Among all age groups, 27 year-olds have the most medical debt on their credit reports.

• *Seniors:* Those on Medicare, unless they have a "Medigap' plan, must pay medical bills from co-pays and out-of-pocket costs, such as some home health care charges. Elders with low or fixed income tend to have unpaid medical bills and high medical debt. Seniors surviving Covid may have the highest medical debt.

> Elders with low or fixed income tend to have unpaid medical bills and high medical debt.

As for home care, an Indiana University study tallied $377 billion in 2017 paid by Medicare and Medicaid, plus $410 billion in "free care" donated by individuals, foundations and corporations. AARP reported in 2018 that about 40 million caregivers provided at least $470 billion in free "hours of service." As the U.S. population ages, there will be fewer and fewer free caregivers, so more debt.

Out of Network Surprises

America's Health Insurance Plans (AHIP), the industry trade group, has found that about 12 percent of all U.S. health claims were for care services obtained from out-of-network providers.

AHIP studied 18 billion claims for the 97 most common health services. People getting treatments from doctors and facilities not covered by insurance plans, said AHIP, received bills from 118 percent to 1,382 percent higher than what Medicare would pay for those same services.

Health Affairs reports almost 20 percent of inpatient hospital admissions that start in the ER lead to unexpected bills. New York's Department of Financial Services told CNBC that surprise bills from out-of-network radiologists in one year averaged $5,406, of which insurers paid on average $2,497. Patients pay the balance.

Find out in advance which providers in your area are in and out of your insurance network. If you live in a rural area, for instance, call now to see if your hospital ER doctors are in your health plan. They likely are not. Their emergency treatments would be deemed out-of-network. Also check anesthesiologists in your area.

Be prepared to specify your in-network provider, if available, for emergency care. Be sure all your emergency contacts have this list of in-network providers, so you better avoid surprise bills.

Laboratory work, in general, is a one big out-of-network bill waiting to happen. Ask your insurer which labs they cover, and demand that all your lab work goes there. Be polite and insistent.

One more critical point: If a doctor ever says, "I'll take whatever your insurance pays," go at once to another doctor because that is illegal. Consider reporting that doctor to state medical authorities. You could get a huge bill you don't expect, a bill you will be legally obliged to pay. Such debt is unfair.

Medicaid in the Debt Terrain

Medical debt mountains are geographically concentrated in the states with limited Medicaid coverage.

AARP interviewed hundreds of people who earned less than $40,000 a year. Nobody on Medicaid had medical debt. In states that expanded Medicaid coverage under ACA (from people earning 100 percent of the poverty level up to 138 percent), we at RIP see fewer requests for debt relief.

Increasing Medicaid coverage from 138 to 200 percent of the poverty level would keep many more people out of medical debt.

In working with AARP, we at RIP learned about a problem for middle-class spouses who need Medicaid to provide services for a loved one. Once the loved one dies, Medicaid stops paying, but the bill keep coming, and debts mount.

It's devastating for me to see a proud, independent person who just lost a spouse suddenly to have all their savings clawed back. This debt mountain stays unseen unless the people buried by debt are willing to climb out, to speak up and be heard.

VA-Covered Veterans

Heaven forbid that a veteran does not pay for any non-covered benefits and winds up owing the VA! The federal government has collection powers that far exceed the enforcement tools of banks or creditors. The "right of offset" gives the government, regardless of hardship or ability to pay, the right to garnish tax refunds to pay off any federal and state liabilities still due.

As for bills veterans owe to the Veterans Health Administration, the government can and will offset not only a tax refund but also monthly benefits. They can offset a medical bill, for example, even if that leaves a veteran with only $25 to live on for the month.

VA members account for more than two million visits every month at non-VA hospitals. Their VA insurance, just like everyone else's insurance, covers only just so much. Veterans too often have limited resources to handle any remaining balance after insurance (BAI). The next step is the bill collector.

RIP is aware of more than $8 billion in medical debt that VA members owe over the last five years from ambulance and ER bills that the VA has denied for payment. We learned this by visiting Washington, DC, and the House Veterans' Subcommittee on Health. We learned that denied VA benefits claims fall to veterans to pay. If not paid, the non-VA ambulance service or hospital must seek collections from the patient or absorb a loss.

Medical debt mountains are concentrated in the states with limited Medicaid.

An audit found that many VA denials are due to inconsistent application of policy and standards. About 90,000 veterans a year are denied coverage due to the VA's "prudent layperson" standard. The VA may use this loose standard to decide, for instance, that an ambulance trip and hospital ER visit was not actually an emergency. These denials save the VA about $3 billion each year while burying our vets in mountains of debt.

Hardship, Poverty, Poor Health

What percentage of Americans experience poverty, poor health or material hardship each year?

The Centers for Disease Control and Prevention (CDC) reports only 7.6 percent of all people in the USA are admitted to the hospital overnight per year. This relatively low use of the healthcare system contributes to a common misperception that medical debt doesn't affect all that many people. Look closer.

According to a three-year study by the Robin Hood Foundation and Columbia University Population Research Center, 63 percent of the residents studied in a community experienced an economic hardship in one year. Specifically, this 63 percent experienced at least one of the defining criteria of being disadvantaged — *poverty, hardship and poor health.*

• *Poverty:* Financial assistance programs assess income levels in determining financial assistance, but "income poverty" can change rapidly just by finding a job. Employment is not enough. About 69 percent of all Americans have less than $1,000 in savings, 49 percent have less than $500, and 34 percent have no savings at all. Those without savings are the most vulnerable to medical debt.

According to a recent Federal Reserve survey, almost 50 percent of all Americans cannot come up with $400 for a sudden medical bill. They would have to sell off an asset or borrow the funds.

Households with medical debt have 70 percent more credit card debt, more debt overall. Sean McElwee in *Demos* reported medically indebted households average $8,762 in credit card debt, this compared to households with $5,154 in credit card debt unrelated to medical bills.

Americans borrow $55 billion per year from friends and family, Olivia Chow reported in *Finder.* Disadvantaged people rarely have friends and family with that kind of money. So, they turn to crowdfunding, where 36 percent of all

> # Almost 50% of all Americans cannot come up with $400 for a sudden medical bill.

money is raised to pay for medical expenses or its residual debt.

> # Medical debt can happen to anyone, any strata or race or gender.

- *Hardship:* The inability to pay your bills is the most persistent disadvantage. For example, the Columbia study found only nine percent of people entering a year in poverty were still in poverty at the end of that year, but 23 percent of those entering a year in material hardship were still there at the end of the year.

- *Poor Health:* Traditional healthcare interventions account for only 20 percent of our health. The other 80 percent is due to factors like physical environment, health behaviors, and socioeconomic conditions. The three main causes of stress are changes in income, work or family dynamics. These three factors drive 75 to 90 percent of all health care visits and related medical debt. Our migration patterns in and out of poverty, hardship and poor health need to be better understood by our healthcare system.

Remove Material Hardship

What if paying for medical bills was not so stressful? What if it did not result in material hardship or financial ruin? What if medical costs did not harm us, our families and our fellow citizens?

Research shows anyone paying more than 2.5 percent of their gross income for out-of-pocket medical bills feels hardship. At least 20 percent of us have hardship medical debt on credit reports.

This means, to relieve suffering, we do not need to completely cancel all medical debt, but we must remove the material hardship caused by it. Reducing hardship to maximize wellbeing is what RIP seeks to do by abolishing unpayable medical — a debt of necessity causing hardship, usually brought on involuntarily by injury, illness or violence. Medical debt is no reason for shame.

Does medical debt forgiveness improve wellbeing? We're about to know this. As I noted, researchers from four universities have undertaken an economic impact study (randomized control trial) of medical debt and debt cancellation. Charitable foundations and policymakers heard preliminary findings in 2020. In 2021, the first of their peer reviewed reports was published in *JAMA,*

What of that other 80 percent of the American people who have not suffered hardship, poor health or poverty? How many feel real empathy for the truly disadvantaged people? Some in the majority may still believe unbidden medical debt is the "fault" of the debtors. The evidence plainly points elsewhere.

Medical debt can happen to anyone, any strata or race or gender. No matter how many assets you may have, even if you think you're well-insured, you are not immune from medical debt.

CHAPTER 4

Insurance is
No Protection

Robert E. Goff

People with health insurance are wise not to feel too secure in their coverage. Insured people are at risk of medical debt.

Employers mitigate their health insurance premium increases by decreasing the employees' coverage and increasing deductibles (amounts paid out-of-pocket before insurance kicks in).

The Kaiser Family Foundation's 2019 Employer Health Benefits Study found that deductibles from 2009 to 2019 rose steeply 162 percent. Adding to economic pressures on families, as the average cost of family coverage topped $20,000 for the first time, employer contributions to that care coverage eroded from 73 percent in 2009 to 70 percent in 2019. In the same time period, workers' earnings rose 26 percent, which for many was not enough.

CNBC reported in 2019 that among people with employer-sponsored insurance, their deductibles increased from 63 percent to 82 percent in the past 10 years. Deductibles have risen from $826 to $1,655, on average.

Worsening the situation is the growth of "High Deductible Health Plans" over the past five years from 18 percent of employed insured to 28 percent. These plans' annual deductibles are at least $1,350 for an individual and $2,000 for a family. The operative term "at least" indicated the base for higher deductibles, which are touted as a way of keeping premiums down.

Lower payroll deductions appeal to people who remain healthy during the year. The cost savings can become a real problem if they get hit by an illness or injury. That's when their economic exposure can be devastating, such as people facing $10,000 deductibles under their plans.

Higher health costs eat more of workers' pay, leaving them exposed to higher bills and more medical debt.

A 2015 Kaiser Family Foundation study found that:

• 62 percent of those stressed by medical bills have insurance.

• 75 percent of those insured say that their insurance co-pays, deductibles, or coinsurance costs are more than they can afford.

• 46 percent of insured workers pay out annual deductibles of $1,000 or more for single-person coverage (up from 41 percent in 2014).

• 39 percent of large firms offering employee health insurance have plans with deductibles of $1,000 or more.

• 20 percent of all those with insurance say paying medical bills caused significant financial disruptions in their lives.

• 11 percent of insured workers end up seeking charity aid.

Simply put, higher healthcare costs are eating more of workers' paychecks, leaving them exposed to higher bills and more medical debt. Covid patients with employer-provided health benefits are not exempt from the high deductibles, co-pays and other limitations of their group insurance plans.

When health insurance is tied to employment, what can keep any working person awake at night is the reality that the coverage he or she has could disappear in the morning with a pink slip. The loss of employment, like from an accident or illness, can quickly move a middle-income family into medically-induced poverty.

That nightmare, reports the Kaiser Family Foundation, by May 2020 became reality for some 27 million Americans who lost their health insurance when they lost their job due to the pandemic. If Covid did not directly cost you your job, the recession could. You may be trying to sleep at night knowing the next reduction in force could include you. That's not what's supposed to happen.

COBRA Costs

In the event of a job loss, federal law protects workers' ability to keep their employer-sponsored health insurance. Under COBRA (Consolidated Omnibus Budget Reconciliation Act), continued health care coverage costs more than when employed.

Under COBRA, a former employee may pay up to 102 percent of the total insurance premium their former employer paid for their coverage. In case of a disability, COBRA coverage can be extended, but at up to 150 percent of the employer's whole premium. They pay what their paid before plus more than the employer's share.

The average annual premium for employer-provided coverage in 2019 was $20,576 for a family, and $7,188 for an individual, according to Kaiser Family Foundation's Annual Employer Health Benefits Report. Faced with a loss of income from lost employment, who can sustain the added pressures on the budget from COBRA? Adding to the disaster, even if you can afford COBRA, coverage is limited to 18 months. After that, too bad, so sad. You're on your own. Go find coverage you can afford.

The designers of COBRA saw coverage as a temporary stop-gap as workers find other jobs with health insurance. No consideration was given to the fact an illness or accident leading to unemployment may preclude re-employment. COBRA mandates the availability of coverage, not affordability, and this assumes a new job has health insurance. Unreal. The Kaiser Family Foundation in 2019 reported only 57 percent of all U.S. employers offer health benefits. The other 43 percent? *Voila!* New candidates for Medicaid.

Fiscal Risks of Hospitalization

Hospitalized patients are among those most victimized by out-of-network situations. The breach may be aided and abetted by the very hospital where they sought professional quality care.

If admitted to a hospital, you are dependent on the institution's care structure. You are reduced to an account number, temporarily occupying a bed, incurring charges. During your hospital stay, you are subject to a fee structure that may put your economic health at risk. Your body may recover, but your finances may not.

Few people realize that hospitals do not control the health plan participation of physicians granted privileges to use the hospital for admitting and treating patients. This applies to most physicians in community hospitals. Even if a hospital hires the physician directly, it may not make sure a new physician employee participates in the same health plans as the hospital, or contracts to accept these plans. In some instances, the hospital for its own business reasons might intentionally not contract for a particular physician or service.

Without you knowing, one or more of your hospital caregivers may not be covered under your plan, such as a physician consulted on your case. *The New Jersey Record* reported an egregious example of a New Jersey hospital that billed a patient $56,980 for a 25-minute bedside consultation from a non-participating physician.

Some hospitals make it worse. They will contract exclusively with physician groups for staffing, but then do not require these physician groups to participate in the hospitals' health plans.

For example, hospitals often contract with physician groups to staff the emergency department or to provide anesthesia services. Physician groups agree to provide 24/7 staffing in trade for exclusive rights to provide those services. However, some hospital may not require these groups to participate in the hospital health plans. They say participation is a group's independent business decision. So, the patients get surprise bills.

Hospitals grant to physician groups excusive monopolies over crucial care services. Monopolies do tend to price monopolistically. The hospital departments most often granted to monopolies are radiology, pathology, anesthesiology, cardio EKG, and ER.

> Some hospitals will contract exclusively with physician groups for their staffing, but then do not require these groups to participate in the hospitals' health plans.

Hospital monopoly groups amply reward the physicians they employ as staff. CNBC in 2016 reported out-of-network emergency room monopoly doctors, on average, were paid 2.7 times more than in-network hospital staff ER doctors were paid for providing the very same exact emergency services.

For patients in economic stress, the hospital may provide some consideration through charity care programs. That charity policy does not necessarily extend to the physician staffing group granted a monopoly by that hospital. The physician group in control of a department of that hospital need not be so considerate. They expect all patients to pay for service rendered.

A community hospital may let contracted physician groups exploit and abuse the community they are licensed to benefit.

The health news program NPR *Shots* in 2019 reported on private ER companies becoming increasingly aggressive in handling long unpaid bills. They filed lawsuits against patients who are poor and near poor.

Explaining the rationale behind aggressive collections, Nashville General Hospital CEO Bruce Naremore told a local NPR reporter in 2019, "It's a private entity that runs the emergency room, and it's the cost of doing business."

He added. "If I restrict them from collecting dollars, then my cost is going to very likely go up, or I'm going to have to find another provider to do it."

I find this system incredible. Hospitals are granted monopolistic licenses by government to benefit the community. Hospital administrators, driven by margin, may abdicate their responsibility to that community for their health and wellbeing.

Community hospitals may let their contracted physician groups exploit and abuse the community they are licensed to benefit. Such a system does not make sense.

Health plans must pay a non-participating physician for care in a life-or-limb emergency visit. Few patients question the insurance participation of the anesthesiologist or radiologist, rarely in elective admissions. If a hospital participates with my insurance, then all the physicians there must participate, too, right? Not necessarily.

Hospitals and physicians are consolidating into "systems" with the avowed benefit that care is coordinated by providers who all are part of one organization. However, a 2014 *Los Angeles Times* article reported that "in system" may not mean "in network." For example, an in-system and yet out-of-network California pathologist charged $81,000 for a tissue exam while Medicare pays only $128.

The Guardian in 2018 told a compelling story about the birth of three sons to Stella Apo Osae-Cwum, insured, who was driven near to bankruptcy by all the out-of-network physician charges at an in-network hospital. She and her husband did it all by the book, used an in-network hospital and obstetrician. When her triplets were born prematurely, a big bill arrived. The hospital's out-of-network neonatologist charged $877,000. Her employer-provided insurance covered most of the bill, but she was responsible for $51,000.

The financial risks to patients while a "captive" of the hospital can be financially stressful, to put it mildly.

Fortunately, the predatory practice of surprise medical billing garnered enough press and political attention that many states have been addressing the situation. Federal legislation was sidetracked by Covid, at first, but then Surprise Billing protections went into the Covid stimulus bill, and these provisions become effective starting January 2022. Until then, it's up to the states to act.

Many patients are still caught up fighting for attention from their insurance company, fighting for protections from what regulations do exist, and doing all this while simultaneously fighting aggressive collection efforts.

The Costs of 'Free' Hospital Care

Some people go to a hospital without paying. Is their care free? According to the American Hospital Association, local hospitals' uncompensated care — including free, discounted, and unpaid care — increased from $35.7 billion in 2015 to $38.3 billion in 2016. The AHA "Uncompensated Care Fact Sheet" reports unpaid care represents 6.2 percent of annual hospital expenses. Hospitals recover lost revenues by "cost-shifting" with higher charges to paying patients, higher charges to health insurers (who increase policy premiums), and from government assistance, paid by our taxes.

Is this system just? Consider the impacts.

An oddity in hospital finance is how uninsured individuals are charged. Patients with insurance are charged the discounted rates negotiated by insurance carriers. Patients without insurance fall into the "self-pay" category. They must fund the full costs of care.

> Uninsured patients are charged the maximum 'self-pay' rates set by the hospital.

Uninsured patients, the least likely to have the means to pay the cost of their care, are charged the maximum self-pay rates set by the hospital. In the hotel business, few guests pay the "rack rate" or full price for a room. The same is true for hospitals.

The pandemic's economic pressures have sharpened the public scrutiny of hospital financing. The American Hospital Association estimated that Covid in 2020 resulted in more than $300 billion in losses for hospitals. The lingering Covid variant losses are projected between $50 billion and $120 billion, and that's conservative.

A hospital's uncompensated care adds to financial pressures on the institution. The most disadvantaged facilities serve communities with the weakest local economies. Hospitals in poor and near-poor areas provide the most unpaid care. Hospital closures caused by unmanageable financial losses happen most often in least well-off communities and neighborhoods.

The ripples from a hospital closure are less access to care, loss of positive economic effects from jobs, making the community less desirable, thereby worsening poverty in the community.

Becker's Hospital Review reports 109 hospitals closed from 2010 to 2018, with 11 closing in 2019. Covid in 2020 pushed another 21 hospitals over a fiscal cliff to closure. All of the acute-care hospitals closing their doors cited financial pressure as a reason, if not *the* reason, for their demise. According to a January 2021 report by the Center for Healthcare Quality and Payment Reform, a staggering 897 U.S. hospitals are at risk of closure.

Most at risk are rural hospitals and urban ones that do not serve large populations of well-insured patients. While medical bad debt is not the sole source of hospitals' fiscal distress, it plainly contributes mightily. As a last resort to avoid closure, hospitals seek bailouts by states and municipalities. That cost is borne by us taxpayers.

The Impact of Healthcare Economics

The cost of health insurance is dependent on the price charged for care, which is based on the cost of care plus a profit margin. Today's medical costs, both legitimate and improper, will become tomorrow's premiums, paid by all.

A physician may participate in a patient's health plan, for example, but then influence a patient to do their procedure at an ambulatory surgery center where the physician has an ownership stake. That non-participating center, unfettered by contract limits, may not hesitate to send a medical bill, a large one. If the bill is not paid, it becomes medical debt.

Medical coverage is tricky. Among the most impactful provisions of insurance coverage are requirements to obtain care "in-network." These provisions make perfect sense from an insurance perspective. In-network providers agree to accept an insurance company's reimbursement rates, and to hold patients harmless should the company go insolvent.

An in-network provider is "credentialed" by the insurance company. They meet the carrier's guidelines for training and licensure. While unusual, some people do practice medicine without any licensure. Far less rare, licensed doctors may practice beyond the scope of their training. Beyond fiscal risks from out-of-network bills, the health risks are why wise patients prefer or demand only in-network providers.

> An in-network provider is 'credentialed' by the insurance company.

Insurance requirements limiting full coverage to in-network care has increasingly put patients in harms way. Even when patients make reasonable efforts to stay in-network, they can find themselves surprised by a bill when coverage is non-existent, or limited, because a treating provider was, in fact, out-of-network.

A non-contracted, out-of-network private ambulatory surgery center in New York used a contracted, participating doctor for a medical procedure, and the surgery center billed a patient $42,000. Insurance would have paid the participating center about $3,000, and the patient's in-network cost would have been just $1,000. This "double jeopardy" meant the physician was paid for professional services and then was paid again separately as an owner of the ambulatory surgery center — enjoying a portion of all the profits earned out-of-network.

Even a conscious patient is at risk going to a physician participating in their health plans. The physician may send a patient's lab specimen to a non-participating laboratory, or refer the patient to a non-participating radiology provider. The unsuspecting patient gets a surprise bill, maybe an outrageous one, when their insurance pays only part of a bill, or else completely denies the claim.

The patient may argue in court that the physician breached their contract by sending the specimen to a non-participating provider. In states with protective "Surprise Billing" laws, patients themselves must initiate civil complaints in their own defense. If patients are unaware of these laws, of course, they cannot access their rightful protections from medical debt.

For unwary patients "captured" by non-participating providers, or by unscrupulous providers, the economic exposures can truly be tremendous. The impacts include a higher deductible, higher cost-sharing, and being held personally responsible for the total bill, the totally outrageous bill.

The Impact on Physicians

Physicians in private practice lack the benefits of a local, state or federal governmental program to offset the impact of bad debt. As patients' debts rise, if a physician is unable to absorb the revenue loss, hard choices must be made. Physicians' responses to excessive medical bad debt, even if ethical, often are unpleasant.

Physicians rarely disengage from a patient over a financial issue. By law and custom, they cannot abandon a patient under their care. If this means providing unpaid care until a patient can find another caregiver, or can be referred away, then so be it.

Patients causing unsustainable financial losses for a physician may be discharged from a medical practice. A discharge also may be self-imposed by a patient, embarrassed to owe for past care, who stops making or keeping appointments. They exile themselves.

The physician, sensitive to a patient's fiscal hardship, may refer a patient to another medical resource, such as a community health center or public clinic. The continuity of care is lost.

Physicians face a stark financial reality. They must earn enough revenue to sustain themselves and their practice. Bad debt rarely can be replaced by raising rates. Physicians' rates are fixed by insurance and government rules. Must doctors absorb a loss for time and resources expended to extend care? Their understandable collection efforts can ruin the physician-patient relationship.

A primary care physician may refer a patient for specialty care. That patient's stressed finances might prompt skipping care or any prescriptions. More ill, the patient returns to primary care, unable to pay bills, or the patient goes to a costly hospital ER.

Medical debt may drive physicians to close practices or relocate for survival, leaving the communities they serve and likely love. Un-collectable patient bills yield uneven distribution of good physicians in our communities, contributing to healthcare deserts. Few physicians locate practices in distressed areas, where the need is greatest, unless fulfilling a duty of their medical education loans.

Some programs forgive physicians' medical school student debt if they agree to practice several years in an underserved community, like an urban clinic or rural hospital. Their service usually is short-term unless lasting bonds form within that community.

The institutions supporting temporary local physicians rely on government financing. Such "supported" medical practices add to the ways medical costs and related debt become financial obligations for the community of taxpayers.

The structure of U.S. medical insurance coverage, under law, virtually assures physicians in private practice have unpaid patient bills. The Affordable Care Act contributed by supporting increased deductibles, today the norm in health benefit coverage.

As deductibles rise higher, the economics of medical attention in a physician's office changes. The patient-physician encounter carries higher fiscal intensity. With $1,000 deductibles or more being increasingly common, the burden of collecting bad debt often lands on the physician. Patient debt can overshadow any office visit.

Reliable data for private physicians' bad debt is hard to locate. Most medical practices use cash-based accounting (record income when received and expenses when paid). Bad debt is not counted as income or expense, so it's missed.

Some studies indicate that bad debt can run between 5.9 percent and 14 percent of any physician's billings. A 2013 Kaiser Family Foundation study found that private office-based physicians provided more than $30 billion in uncompensated care. That surely is higher today.

The structure of U.S. medical insurance coverage, under law, virtually assures physicians in private practice have unpaid patient bills. The Affordable Care Act contributed by supporting increased deductibles.

If a physician closes an office due to bad debt, the patients suffer disruption of care, possibly harming their health.

Perhaps worse, the community loses a caregiver.

If the physician closes their practice to become an employee of a hospital, for patients who follow them, their billing mirrors that of the hospital. The employed physician is disallowed from extending time to patients they know suffer physically and economically.

As staff physicians rely more on costly hospital-based ancillary services, rarely using independent local providers like radiologist, even in-network costs increase. Independent community providers lose patients, adding to the economic pressures. As practices close their doors, community care services shrink. With less competition, hospital and physician group fees may rise, reducing care access for the uninsured. The impact spreads outward into society.

Uncollectable patient bills yield uneven distribution of physicians in communities, contributing to healthcare deserts.

Covid appears to have accelerated the declining availability and supply of physicians in private practice. Stress from Covid reportedly motivated thousands of practices to close as physicians sought the shelter of hospital employment, or else they retired.

Like other small businesses, medical practices temporally closed or reduced hours of operations. A survey by the Medical Society of New York State reported that 82 percent of practices had experienced a reduction of at least 50 percent of their patent volume since the pandemic began.

Without a large organization like a hospital or medical group to help absorb the revenue loss, the private physicians, long seen as part of the economic elite, are now among those suffering.

The Impact on Patients

The ACA was supposed to solve health care issues by removing financial status as a barrier to obtaining medical care. It didn't work. Medical insecurity continues as Congressional and court activities put the ACA benefits in doubt, such as full coverage for preexisting conditions, for preventive care without co-pays or deductibles.

The ACA's failure to cut the costs of delivering care contributes to the upward spiral of premiums, translating into higher payroll dedications or higher deductibles. More than ever now, ACA theory and reality do not match.

If health is restored and people can return to the workforce with paid insurance, they remain liable for all accumulated prior debt. To pay off old bills, they often skip or skimp on needed medication and follow-up care. This is especially true (and most troubling) for those with chronic debilitating diseases, such as diabetes, where skipping treatment can rapidly deteriorate health, resulting in far higher care bills.

> ACA theory and reality do not match.

Not filling a prescription can be costly and deadly. ProMed.gov compared patients who follow instructions to those who don't take medications as intended, including for financial reasons. They risk hospitalization, re-hospitalization and premature death 5.4 times higher in cases of hypertension, 2.8 times higher with dyslipidemia, and 1.5 times higher in cases of heart disease.

"Putting it off" is no solution.

Studies report people who delay or forego care are less likely to report "very good" or "excellent" health. They have lower quality-of-life scores compared to those who don't delay necessary medical care. This cost of delayed care can be confirmed. Study the impact of Covid on patients and their care. Patients afraid of Covid exposure deferred their care, but Covid then made such care unavailable, causing an increase in community fatality rates up to 10 percent.

> Patients afraid of high bills might not take advantage of a hallmark ACA benefit — coverage for preventive care without deductibles.

I respect a 2013 University of Chicago and AP survey, "Privately Insured in America: Opinions on Health Care Costs and Coverage." Among adults ages 18 to 64 with commercial insurance, 19 percent did not visit a doctor when ill, and 18 percent skipped recommended preventive care.

Personal responsibility is not universal.

An unfortunate impact of all the byzantine rules for coverage is patients' confusion on benefits and concern for costs, deterring them from early detection and treatment of their ailments. Patients afraid of high bills might not take advantage of a hallmark ACA benefit — coverage for preventive care without deductibles.

As the classic example, if you skip a cancer screening, believing you'd have to pay a sizable deductible, perceived short-term savings from skipping the screening may yield a later identification of more advanced cancer. If cancer is identified too late for successful treatment, you may pay for delay with your life.

Not understanding your health plan benefits means exposure to higher costs, or missing out on benefits to help retain your health. I believe "health illiteracy" — the lack of understanding one's health coverage — is too rampant. Even when wise enough to seek medical treatment, the fact of not being able to pay the medical bills creates its own set of challenges.

A 2015 Kaiser Family Foundation study identified nationwide averages for the ways people handle high costs for medical care:

- 77 percent cut spending for household purchases or vacations.
- 63 percent use up most or all of their savings.
- 42 percent take an extra job or work more hours.
- 38 percent increase their credit card debt or max out the cards.
- 37 percent borrow money from family or friends.
- 14 percent change their living situations.

Even with insurance, millions of Americans are living only one accident or illness away from potential financial disaster. Could you and your family handle a serious illness or injury?

Medical debt from medical care is the great economic equalizer. According to Kaiser, about 44 percent of the people with employer-based health insurance paying medical bills shared nearly identical consequences as the 45 percent paying for their health care without insurance. Does high-deductible insurance beat self-pay?

Medical debt is an equal opportunity destroyer.

The weak can never forgive.
Forgiveness is the attribute of the strong.

— MAHATMA GANDHI

CHAPTER 5

No Thank You for
Your Service

Jerry Ashton

In November 2017, for the first time in more than 50 years, I put on my mothballed Navy uniform to march in the New York City Veterans Day Parade. I was joined by Mikel Burroughs, a retired Army colonel and Director of Military Debt Acquisitions and Relief at RIP, and by Hutch Dubosque, a Vietnam-era Army sergeant and battlefield medic who advises our organization.

We were there to represent RIP and bring more attention to the unpayable medical bills of veterans and active-duty military.

As I marched in uniform that day, bystanders said, "Thank you for your service!" I appreciated acknowledgment of the four years I served as a U.S. Navy journalist. Even so, I heard these words with mixed emotions. Should I be thanked for service I gave decades earlier? How did that "thank you" translate into reality?

On reflection, I felt compelled to write a *Huffington Post* piece suggesting that Americans replace the words, "Thank you for your service," with something more tangible and action-oriented. This was my polite way to suggest that any person shaking a military or veteran's hand could express a more useful form of gratitude — forgiving their medical debt!

This unusual possibility had been created years earlier when in 2014 Craig Antico and I along with Robert E. Goff founded RIP Medical Debt as a tax-deductible way for people to help us locate, buy and forgive medical debt burden. As we bought debt portfolios, we found a surprising percentage of medical bills were for veterans, also active-duty military. It struck us that in addition to helping the general population, we must work to forgive debt for our veterans. (Craig's passion for this is evident in his Chapter 3.)

A referral led me to Mikel Burroughs. Mikel (pronounced like "Michael") served as an Army brigade commander in Kuwait and Iraq, retiring as a bird colonel. He'd become a C-suite collections industry executive who'd bought and sold billions in medical debt. He felt strongly about forgiving medical debt and making life easier for his fellow veterans. A perfect fit for RIP.

With Mikel on the team, we launched a campaign devoted to abolishing medical debt for veterans. We reached our 2018 goal of forgiving $50 million in veterans' debt, and by 2021 passed $100 million, which is still barely a drop in the debt ocean.

I believe America is failing in its role of protecting and healing its military family. In recent years, the systemic ills seem to have worsened. How can a nation fervently claiming to value its warriors let the egregious emotional and financial wounding of unpayable medical debt be inflicted upon veterans year after year?

The least objectionable explanation may be that too few people in the general public understand the healthcare problems faced by veterans. Another explanation may be that too many people simply do not sympathize with veterans, particularly when it comes to vets' economic struggles to pay medical bills.

Only since the consciousness-raising advent of Covid ha most Americans become alert to the economic affects of impossible-to-pay bills and unresponsive healthcare administrators. Now that the medical debt problem has been so personalized by Covid, civilians and veterans are more conjoined.

The financial pressure on veterans from medical debt contributes to hopelessness, depression and suicide. The VA's National Suicide Data Report analyzed veteran suicide data for all 50 states and the District of Columbia from 2005 to 2015. This report found an average of 20 veteran suicides a day remained unchanged over the decade. The suicide rate increased faster among the vets who seldom or never used the Veterans Health Administration care plan, as compared to suicides among vets who sought VA care coverage.

> The financial pressure on veterans from medical debt contributes to hopelessness, depression and suicide.

Fortunately, we are seeing a shift in how average Americans handle personal issues, like a top Olympic athlete taking a mental health timeout. People across the spectrum are now more willing to voice their grievances, but few vets seek attention. Some may reveal their challenges to friends and loved ones, but seldom with the press.

Twentieth century veterans often reentered the population with little complaint. Recent veterans of Middle East fights do the same. The uniforms pulled from storage for Memorial Day and Veterans Day are quietly put away again. Veterans' claim for public attention to their problems is tucked away along with their uniforms.

Yes, Vets Do Have Medical Debt

You may be asking, how can anybody in the service (active-duty or veteran) have medical debt? What about Veterans Affairs (VA) and the Veterans Benefits Administration?

When military men and women enter the service, they basically sign a blank check saying, "I'm yours to use as needed, America, up to and including sacrificing my life," Decade after decade, America cashes that check — sometimes in full. When vets try to cash their check at the VA for illnesses or injuries, too often it bounces.

Like most Americans (even myself as a veteran), I was under the impression that our country covers all the medical needs of men and women who serve or have served our country. Many return from deployment suffering severe disabilities. Some wounds are visible; others are not. Surely, our nation would tend to our warriors' needs as our share of the bargain? Not exactly.

There is no truth to this common misperception that troops and veterans are entitled to free health care for life. Health care benefits for military members, retirees and their families are and have always been "as provided by law." That law provides free medical care for service members and their families on active duty. IF you have a service-related disability during your tour or after, and IF you meet set income requirements, you *may* be eligible for lifetime medical care. But first you have to jump through a series of hoops.

Consider the complex regulations a veteran must understand and obey to obtain medical care at the VA.

Until recently, the VA largely refused to cover vets for off-site care by non-military physicians, clinics and hospitals. Worse, the VA would not cover charges for emergency transportation and care by an ambulance. "Uncle Sugar" has rejected literally billions of dollars in such claims over this past decade.

That may be changing.

A federal court ruled in 2019 that the government is required to reimburse such claims. The court declared that Veterans Affairs has improperly denied reimbursements for care at non-VA facilities not covered by private insurance. This was the second time since 2015 a court overruled the VA's interpretation of how veterans should be reimbursed on emergency claims. The latest ruling may cost the VA $1.5 to $6.5 billion in reimbursements for hundreds of thousands of vets with claims pending since 2016.

Consider the shocking statistics: Approximately eight percent of the U.S. population comprises veterans, and half of all these use VA services. About 20 veterans a day commit suicide. Close to 40,000 homeless veterans seek shelter nightly. More than 50 percent of returning vets suffer from PTSD. Many vets discover their long-term health care needs outlast their VA benefits.

> Many vets discover their long-term health care needs outlast their VA benefits.

Sen. Bob Casey (D-CA) on the Finance Committee reported that 30 percent of returning vets, aged 18 to 24, are unprepared to cope with personal finance, low-paying jobs and unemployment. Regardless of a willingness to protect America, they lack the resources and reserves to handle financial adversity.

Almost 50 percent of the 20 million U.S. veterans participate in the labor force, which leaves more than 10 million veterans either not working or else not actively looking for work. Some veterans are retired or on disability. Some may be in school. Some have given up on ever finding a job.

A 2020 study by Bob Woodruff Foundation showed 14 percent of the veteran workforce is employed in industries most pressured by Covid to lay off or furlough employees. The report found nearly 500,000 vets live in 15 cities "most likely to face significant impacts as a result of these industrial downturns,"

As for the millions of working veterans whose health insurance is tied to their jobs, they remain at high risk of medical debt. If the job goes for any reason their insurance goes. In 2015, thanks to the ACA, the number of uninsured veterans dropped by 40 percent — down to 429,000. Even with ACA, out-of-pocket costs often outstrip disposable income, which leads to unpaid bills and collections.

The leading federal agency protecting health consumers from unfair collection practices is the Consumer Financial Protection Bureau (CFPB), briefly renamed by a Trump Administrator as the Bureau of Consumer Financial Protection. Half the complaints CFPB got from service members in 2015, reported Herb Weisbaum at NBC News, dealt with "being hounding to pay medical bills that should have been covered by insurance" (the VA, Medicare, Medicaid, or private insurance). CFPB says veterans file twice the level of federal consumer complaints about debt collectors as the general public.

> # Consumer Financial Protection Bureau says veterans file twice the level of federal consumer complaints about debt collectors as the general public.

Active duty military, by comparison, including those in the reserves, actually are more easily pressured by bill collectors to pay an outstanding medical bill, even if it's not still owed or not correct. They worry that the collection agency could (illegally) contact their commanding officer, hurting their military career, which is not so for vets. They also fear, as do veterans, that a collection agency may (legally) place a bad mark on their credit report, hindering their financial future and the wellbeing of their family.

No matter what pleas for flexibility that vets and military make to an aggressive or even predatory collection agency, these "debtors" are treated as turnips from which blood must be squeezed. The calls and letters from collectors never stop.

As if debt collection pressure was not bad enough, along came Covid-19. The VA in October 2020 reported by then they had tested 846,889 veterans and employees for Covid, diagnosing 63,966 with the virus. Some 13,000 were in VA facilities, and 55,032 had reached convalescence. The National Cemetery Administration, responsible for military cemeteries, reported that 3,501 of 82,367 internments (burials) were Covid-related.

The Bob Woodruff Foundation issued a 2020 paper analyzing the pandemic-related needs of the veteran community. It detailed the potential acute and long-term impacts, including mental health challenges and economic concerns of our vets — "the first to volunteer and the last to ask for help." My rough summary:

1. Vast numbers of veterans are likely to become unemployed at the highest rates since post-9/11.

2. A "perfect storm" of traumatic loneliness from social isolation and lost income threatens the mental health of many veterans.

3. New veterans transitioning from the military into civilian life (200,000 to 250,000 annually), especially if older in years, suffer the most from unemployment and job loss.

4. Younger veterans have limited savings, insufficient to support them through unemployment lasting longer than six months.

Veteran medical debt is real and has real consequences. We long for the day that RIP secures enough donations and greater access to VA medical debt, so we can help lift this burden totally from those who've faithfully served our nation.

As illustrations, below are four wrenching examples of veterans with medical debt who struggle under the existing VA system.

The Case of 'Veteran Alpha'

In late 2018, I was referred by a friend to a 73-year-old disabled American veteran (DAV) who deserved medical debt forgiveness. He clearly fit our profile, but RIP cannot single out any individual for help because we buy unpaid debt in bulk. Making it harder to help him, our charity had no access to any records of VA-generated debt. I felt regret that we could not help him.

The man's story resonated with me. His travails struck me as a classic cautionary tale of what happens when illusion meets reality. People believe Veterans Affairs takes care of vets' medical bills, but the VA in too many cases fails miserably in its mission.

Believing America would benefit by knowing his story, I worked for months persuading him to go public. Proud and independent like most vets, he's finally allowed this write-up in hope of helping to change the policies and practices of the Veterans Administration. He agreed only on the form condition that I protect his identify, so he stays anonymous.

"Veteran Alpha," as I named him, was barely treading water. He suffered many hardships in struggling to pay hospital bills deemed non-reimbursable by the VA.

The financial tragedies began when he followed the ambulance that was taking his wife to the ER in critical condition from a broken hip and leg. While waiting in the ER, he was approached by a nurse who said he appeared ro be in severe physical and mental distress. He'd been given a clean bill of health a week ago by his VA cardiologist, so he politely declined her offer of help.

Within minutes, she returned and said he really needed to be seen, and "right NOW!"

He was placed in a wheelchair, hustled off for an MRI and EKG, and returned to the ER, where his wife was still being treated. Soon after, the hospital's chief cardiac surgeon arrived to advise him that he needed an immediate double-bypass operation. His primary heart artery and two others were severely blocked. How could this be? Just nine days before at a VA hospital, he'd passed an induced stress test, EKG and CT scan. The doctor pronounced he was "in excellent condition,"

Now he was shocked.

Veteran Alpha was wheeled to his wife's bedside, where the doctor explained the diagnosis and his urgent need for surgery. She agreed. He agreed.

> Per protocol, the ER called the nearest VA medical center, 75 miles away, to get their permission to do emergency surgery. The VA refused.

As he waited in a separate ER room, the physician learned of his retired DAV military status. Per protocol, the ER called the nearest VA medical center, 75 miles away, to report his condition and get their permission to do emergency surgery. The VA refused.

Instead, they VA center said they would send an ambulance in Friday night traffic to transport him to their location. Veteran Alpha sat listening to the back-and-forth. He heard the ER physician agree to the transport. Seemed to him that money and expense was the VA's first priority, not his life.

Veteran Alpha told me the ER physician and his hospital likely were glad to hand him off to the VA and avoid trying to get reimbursed by the VA under the "Veterans Choice Program," famous for its "no pay or slow-pay" reputation. (The program has since been discontinued.)

He was caught in a tragic trap of the VA's misdiagnosis and its non-paying 'Choice' program.

As Veteran Alpha put it, he was caught in a tragic trap of the VA's misdiagnosis and its non-paying Choice program.

At that point, Alpha was put on the phone with the VA center clerk, who questioned him about making his choice of where to be treated. He groggily told the clerk he was in no condition to be transported. He was at extremely high risk of another heart episode, maybe a final one. He said the civilian hospital was already prepping him for emergency surgery.

His options became clear when the clerk said they were "full up" but would do their best to get him into a room. Essentially, he had decided under pressure whether in stay where he was and live, or be transported to the VA and possibly die.

He told the VA clerk, "I have no choice."

He ended the call and went under the knife.

After surviving heart surgery, Veteran Alpha suffered the next indignity. He was swamped with medical bills because the VA, as usual, refused to pay the civilian hospital that saved his life. Why the refusal? He had refused the VA's offer of emergency transport.

His hospital bills for surgery totaled well over $180,000, not including post-op care and initial ambulance charges for his wife. Medicare covered about 80 percent. Because they could not afford a Medicare supplemental plan, soon after the VA refused to pay the balance, the hospital pursued his due 20 percent co-pay. A balance of $36,000 was his "patient responsibility."

Veteran Alpha and his wife emptied their savings accounts and borrowed from a credit union, but he still owed $15,000. In failing health, living on service-related disability income, he's been fighting the system ever since. By the time we met, he has reached the point of believing the VA is essentially "malevolent."

He told me, "I'd been a DAV Service Officer for countless years and thought I'd seen every rotten trick in the book. I was wrong. In my own case, as in so many others, the VA was callous, reckless with mis-diagnosed treatments, unsympathetic and inattentive. This has caused tremendous physical and financial hardship along with cruel mental duress for me and my wife."

He particularly directed his anger at the failed Veterans Choice Program. When he spoke about the time consuming approvals and the paperwork required, more anger poured out. "These roadblocks to my treatment are better known as 'Case Load Backup' caused by the lack of congressional funding, lack of trained personnel, CYA tactics, and wrongful denials of legal and promised appeals."

He bemoaned to me about always hearing from VA clerks the same soul-piercing by-the-manual statement, "We received your claim and are working on it." In his view, they never did.

Veteran Alpha described his post-op condition — exacerbated by "intense collection threats" — as something that he and his wife can no longer endure. "We are old, tired and still in pain, with very little fight or hopeful prospects left. If there ever was a time for the support troops to show up, it's now."

Liver Fluke Cancer and the VA

Hutch DuBosque has been waging a fight to secure formal VA acknowledgment, testing and treatment for service-related bile duct and liver cancers caused by a six known parasites grouped under the name, *platyhelminthes*. His fight reminds me of the long campaign for VA recognition of Agent Orange.

In 2016, several of Hutch's Vietnam-era vet friends came down with a "weird disease" from an obscure parasite — a "liver fluke." As two of the men were dying, Hutch and his four surviving friends promised to research this disease and save others vets' lives. They volunteered for a rescue mission.

The river fluke, according to the American Cancer Society, is a freshwater-borne flatworm found in military men and women who served in eastern and southeastern Asia. It produces a protein called "granulum" — highly carcinogenic. If caught in its dormancy, the parasite is treatable. If not discovered, it inevitably presents as Stage 4 cancer in the pancreas or liver. As Hutch describes it, "Basically, an advanced river fluke diagnosis is a death sentence."

Hutch say the VA will not even test for the parasite or granulum on the grounds that "it's not been proven." It's a Catch 22. Without testing there is no way to determine if a vet has the parasite. Since there is no evidence, there is no point in testing.

The VA claimed they don't have a test, anyway. In actual fact, Hutch says, a lab in South Korea, where the liver fluke is native, has such a test. The FDA is aware of the Asian lab's testing capability and reliability. The VA seems unaware. He asks, "Do any of these agencies ever talk to each other? If not, why not?"

Hutch and four of his friends (John Ball, Gerry Wiggins, Larry Noon, and Ralph Goodwin) volunteered for a 50-person pilot study by the VA Medical Center at Northport, NY. Veterans who reported eating undercooked freshwater fish while in Vietnam donated blood samples for serological exam at Seoul National University College of Medicine in South Korea.

Norfolk's study was published in January 2018 by *Infectious Diseases in Clinical Practice*. The report is entitled, "Screening U.S. Vietnam Veterans for Liver Fluke Exposure 5 Decades After the End of the War." Researchers found that among the 50 Vietnam veterans tested, one in four harbored the parasite, which can live dormant in a body for decades.

The findings were discounted by the VA for having only 50 people in the study sample. Hutch laments, "They have stonewalled the issue ever since we brought it to their attention,"

Hutch and his friends were interviewed by the Long Island newspaper, *Newsday*, for a story about the Norfolk study. The story reported that since 2013, the VA had received 240 claims for bile duct cancers attributed to the liver fluke parasite, and the VA had "rejected more than 76 percent of those claims."

The five Long Island veterans next reached out to Sen. Chuck Schumer (D-NY) and Rep. Tom Suozzi (D-NY), who called for a broader study, still not done.

> It's a Catch 22. VA will not test for the parasite because 'It's not been proven.' Without testing there is no way to determine if a veteran has the parasite. Since there is no evidence, there is no point in testing.

Fast forward to 2021. Hutch's is still pushing for the VA to pay vets' river fluke cancer claims.

He says now that although nobody has proven for certain that any vet acquired the liver fluke while serving in Asia, "this disease affects three times more vets than Agent Orange, but its victims are systematically being denied disability claims by the VA."

During the Vietnam War era and since, three million GIs have served in Indochina, including the U.S. troops today serving in the parasite's range, especially South Korea. Neither the VA nor the Department of Defense routinely screens for the parasite.

"The VA has gaslighted all efforts on liver fluke cancer," Hutch protests. "They keep responding with the same old 'We're in the process' answer that they gave us six years ago."

'The VA has gaslighted all efforts on liver fluke cancer.'

Hutch and his buddies have all tested positive for bile duct cancer. In 2018, he had cancerous cysts removed from his bile duct at Memorial Sloan Kettering Cancer Center. He's now following up with annual CT scans to monitor. For him and his friends, given millions still at risk, their rescue mission continues. Their promise has not yet been kept.

Legislatively, as of this writing, the only federal bills aimed at funding a scientifically valid research study, the "Vietnam Veterans Liver Fluke Cancer Study Act," was introduced in the 115th Congress by Rep. Lee Zeldin (R-NY). The bill died in the House with no co-sponsors and without action taken, not even assignment it to a committee. Zeldin then reintroduced the bill in the 116th Congress, where nothing happened, and again in the current 117 Congress (H.R. 1273), and still no action has been taken.

Hutch and his friends have been told, essentially, that to get any traction in Congress, they personally need to get co-sponsors for the bill, possibly going around the country to drum up local vet support. This is beyond the means of these five aging vets on fixed incomes. And so the bill languishes.

In my view, once again, an unequal and unnecessary burden is being placed upon the backs of our veterans with service-related ailments and injuries.

"No thank you for your service."

Veteran Debt Prevents Transplant

I recently became alert to the struggles of disabled Army cavalry scout and combat medic Michael Thorin, now a medically retired firefighter and paramedic, suffering from "Constrictive Broncioloitis Obliterans and Reactive Airway Dysfunction Syndrome." He's seeking a lung transplant.

The key barrier preventing that transplant from happening is an unpaid medical debt produced by the VA in 2018 rejecting their responsibility to pay for surgical services rendered at the University of Alabama (UAB) hospital, which is across the street from the local VA Medical Center (VAMC) in Birmingham.

At the time, VAMC staff members assured him the bill would be paid, but the VA administrators disagreed, citing chapter and verse. Michael was told that (a) UAB was not an authorized VA provider, and (b) he did not go through the VA for the referral. The $3,000 bill was deemed his responsibility. This was despite the fact Michael's specialist at the VA provided proper paperwork setting up the UAB surgery, which was unavailable at the Birmingham VAMC.

That $3,000 university hospital bill was unpayable, and it still is. Before long, calls and letters began coming from a collection agency, and these continue through today. He's on a thin edge.

Is this just another example of things slipping through the VA cracks? Is Michael merely another veteran not being responsible or aware or medically qualified enough to evade his health problems? Hardly. He is a veteran, due to a series of severe illnesses resulting from combat service in Iraq, who lost his job and career as a firefighter and paramedic, now only subsisting on disability income.

> # He can't afford going to the private sector for a lung transplant, so now it's a race between the VA and the grim reaper.

This all came about after three years struggling with the VA for recognition and treatment for a lung condition that developed on his last 2006 deployment to Iraq . The disease, called *tracheobronchomalaci*, causes airways to narrow, get weak and collapse.

Michael today lives with one lung functioning at 45 percent capacity, the other at 25 percent. When I first connected with him, one lung was at 50 percent, the other at 35 percent. He's waiting for the VA to schedule him for a transplant. He can't afford going to the private sector for a transplant, so now it's a race between the VA and the grim reaper.

He's worked with Alabama's attorney general, secretary of state and congressman to obtain VA approval for a lung transplant. He's informed by all that nothing can happen under VA rules until his outstanding bill at UAB is paid. He lacks the means.

It took many phone calls and emails before Michael agreed to share his story. Getting veterans to volunteer information on their medical debt hardships is not easy. Even if they don't feel shame for being sick, they feel shamed from being broke and chased by bill collectors. Michael does not expect telling his tale will change anything in his life or circumstances. He hopes his tale helps change the VA system for the sake of their veterans. He wrote to me:

> Thousands of Persian Gulf vets like me are caught up in the red tape of a system with skilled and dedicated doctors and nurses working under it, but who work in a system that seems designed to cause confusion more than foster health and healing.
>
> What I want is that my life has not been lived in vain. My wife and kids watch me grow weaker. My grandkids will only hear stories about the man I used to be. They've never seen me strong and healthy. They've never seen me without a tank of oxygen by my side. My story may help others, but only if the right people hear it."

Are you that right person? Our government has told this veteran in no uncertain terms, "No thank you for your service."

Veteran Debt from Burn Pits

Late in 2017, I connected with retired U.S. Army Lt. Col. Robert "Bob" Bent, an activist member of the Disabled American Veterans organization. He became a good friend and a strong proponent of the work we do at RIP in locating and abolishing medical debt for veterans and active military.

Part of his support was showing up at a 2019 event that RIP held in Washington, DC, called, "An Evening to End Medical Debt." He spoke about the importance of enacting legislation to protect vets from the economic scourge of unpayable healthcare bills.

We circled back in early 2020 to put together a draft resolution for his Virginia DAV chapter to present to the state organization for approved to present for national consideration at the summertime

DAV convention in Dallas. If adopted, the resolution would become part of DAV's formal Congressional legislative agenda for 2020 into 2021. Covid canceled the Virginia and national DAV conventions in 2020. The legislative proposal is being resubmitted for adoption at upcoming conventions.

This effort by veterans for veterans could one day create congressional enactment of a law to mitigate our veterans being put at financial risk for medical and economic circumstances beyond their control or financial capability to handle.

To show what's possible in Congress, let me share a 2018 email to our website: "I realize that you buy bundles of old debt, so debt forgiveness is random, and you can't help individuals. But us burn pit veterans get short shrift. We don't get real help from the VA. I have not found any fund that helps burn pit veterans afford medications or inhalers or oxygen to benefit their daily living."

Unaware of "burn pits," I began doing research.

The Department of Veterans Affairs defines a "burn pit" as the common way the military has disposed of waste at military sites in Middle East war zones. They burned chemicals, paint, medical and human waste, munitions, and unexploded ordinance — just about everything combustible went into a burn pit, fouling the air. I found only anecdotal reports of burning tires as fuel.

Mounting evidence indicated that military personnel and contractors working at or near burn pits were suffering from excessive lung diseases, Growing concerns in 2014 led the VA to launch the "Airborne Hazards and Open Burn Pit Registry."

A referral led me to the D.C. offices of U.S. Rep. Raul Ruiz (D-CA), himself a physician. "Burn pits absolutely are a major concern," he declared, "and I'm doing something about it."

Dr. Ruiz in 2018 launched the bipartisan Congressional Burn Pits Caucus, co-chaired by Brad Wenstrup (R-OH), then chair of the House Veterans' Affairs subcommittee, starting with 21 caucus members. The "Helping Veterans Exposed to Burn Pits Act" became U.S. law that year. The VA is now directed to establish a center of excellence in the prevention, diagnosis, mitigation, treatment, and rehabilitation of health conditions relating to exposure to burn pits pollution and other environmental exposures in Afghanistan or Iraq or elsewhere, any burn pit anywhere, as I understand it.

He next successfully added to the 2019 National Defense Authorization Act (NDAA) measures requiring the Department of Defense (DOD) to do a feasibility study on phasing out open burn pits along with conducting annual education campaigns on eligibility for the burn pits registry.

> The 2021 Burn Pit Registry Enhancement Act recognizes 12 pulmonary diseases.

Rep. Ruiz later introduced the Jennifer Kepner HOPE Act for burn pit veterans to be eligible for VA Priority Group 6 health care. He also introduced the Veterans' Right to Breathe Act,,which would establish a VA presumption of service-connected exposure to burn pits for nine specific pulmonary diseases, including asthma, pneumonia, and chronic bronchiolitis. Sadly, the bill did not become law, but his other bill have.

The 2020 NDAA signed by Trump enacted his bills directing the DOD to implement a plan to phase out nine active burn pits identified by Congress. Another directs the DOD to give Congress and the VA a full list of all military bases, posts, outposts, and locations where open-air burn pits have been used. Comedian Jon Stewart lent a hand by calling public attention to the burn pits issue.

The 2021 NDAA signed by Biden includes his Burn Pit Registry Enhancement Act, which (among other things) expands the registry to 12 pulmonary diseases.

Due to Dr. Ruiz and his bipartisan colleagues in the House and Senate, veterans and active duty military now have far less exposure to medical debt resulting from their exposure to burn pits.

Now that is real help! Yes, thank you for your service.

Let me put into context his success getting the VA to recognize and pay for any service-related illness. If Congress and the Department of Veterans Affairs accept responsibility for covering veterans with burn pits ailments, as they did with Agent Orange, I find cause to feel hope that Congress and the VA — given enough popular support and political will — can accept responsibility for relieving the unpayable medical debt burdens of veterans and active-duty military willing to sacrifice their lives for our nation.

Charity for Veterans

The problem is not that individual Americans don't care about veterans. Overwhelmingly, they do. Of some 1.5 million nonprofit organizations in the USA, GuideStar estimates 45,000 nonprofits are devoted to veterans and their families.

These organizations come in every stripe and color, according to a CNBC report on the "Top 10 Charities That Support Veterans." Some were formed by military wives or focus on specific branches of the service. For instance, one charity, Puppies Behind Bars, trains prison inmates to raise service dogs for wounded war veterans. Only 18 percent of all these organizations are 501(c)(3) charities that can accept tax-deductible contributions (like RIP).

Organizations that most Americans recognize are the Veterans of Foreign Wars (VFW) and Disabled American Veterans (DAV). A "newcomer" is Wounded Warriors, begun in 2003 by a group of

Virginia veterans and their friends who chose to take action to help injured service men and women. (RIP is available to help any such organization — military or civilian — raise funds to abolish unpaid and unpayable medical bills for military and veterans.)

After Veterans Day, What?

Every year after Veterans Day, after the flags are furled, after the marching bands return home, after we've duly acknowledged the 20 million men and women alive today who have served their nation, what do we Americans do? In my view, we don't do much, and what we do is not enough.

If you are similar to most Americans, you might take time each Memorial Day to honor those who have fought and still fight for our country. Perhaps you stand to watch or join a parade in the smallest towns to the largest cities across the country. More likely, you watch a parade snippet on the evening news after discount buying in a shopping mall (if Covid allows). Sadder, maybe the day passes by without you noticing or giving veterans a thought.

> After Veterans Day, the vets we thank for their service are still here, as are their medical bills.

The attention America pays to veterans tends to fade after Veterans Day and Memorial Day. Vets starve for attention the other 363 days of the year.

The parades are over. The cemetery salutes are done. Yet, the veterans we thank for their service are still here — as are their medical bills.

I belive we can find a better way to value them.

The main thing I remembered from my high school civics class is that "we the people" are the government. What are we going to do about this blight on our national character? Perhaps veterans and civilians, working together, can remove the emptiness of "Thank you for your service."

I've only pointed to the tip of the veterans' medical debt iceberg, showing a few symptoms of systemic problems. The system creating "vet med debt" exists at the highest levels of government.

At worst, I've decided, our VA officials are cold and uncaring. At best, they're doing what they can despite complex bureaucracies and insufficient funding.

I know that RIP wants Veterans Affairs to grant access to their unpaid medical receivables. If the VA makes available the accounts in hardship for purchase by our charity, we will learn as will the public, the full financial and emotional impact of veterans' medical debt. So, I urge opening the VA digital and actual filing cabinets to make overdue vet accounts available for debt forgiveness.

Burdening our veterans with medical debt is not a way to thank them for their service.

CHAPTER 6

Margin Over Mission: Head vs. Heart

Robert E. Goff

The healthcare industry is a huge part of the American economy. Along with spending on services, the healthcare industry is the largest source of employment in the nation.

All the trillions spent on healthcare are spread across numerous enterprises, yet it's concentrated in two components — physicians and hospitals. The American Medical Association reports these two represent just under half of all healthcare spending.

Hospitals are familiar as all those large, imposing buildings that have been here forever, fixtures in our communities. Physicians are honored for their knowledge and compassion. Each is expected to be a reincarnation of Marcus Welby, MD.

While we think of them as linked, hospitals and physicians are different and separate economic units. How each is compensated has determined how they've evolved, and how they evolved greatly impacts healthcare costs. All of these costs, outstripping the ability of patients to pay, are what create medical debt.

The Urge to Merge

Consolidating economic power is increasing medical costs.

The structure of healthcare delivery is a vestige of 19th and 20th century concepts and limits. If care required more than a physician, the hospital played a critical role as a hub of sophisticated services and technology, such as surgical services, radiology and laboratory. Before immunizations, hospitals also protected communities from communicable diseases.

Hospitals continued in this humble role while the world around them changed. Isolated communities were then linked by roads and bridges. Populations shifted to greener pastures and then the cities. Advances in medical science and technologies reduced the need for hospitals' most critical service — inpatient beds.

Hospitals survived by adapting, if they could. Between 1975 and 2020, about 1,500 hospitals closed their doors. Eliminating beds and hospitals did not slow spending. Statista reported hospital expenditures rose from $27.2 billion in 1980 to over $1.32 trillion in 2020, which is 30 percent of the total healthcare expenditures.

The American hospital has evolved from a community charity with a mission of service into a business enterprise. Hospitals were licensed by governments to guarantee competence in assuring that minimal standards were met for safety and the quality of care. The license to operate let hospitals become monopolies or oligarchies in their service areas.

Historically, licensed local hospitals used business techniques to control how the healthcare dollar was spent in their communities. Their license let them dominate inpatient hospital services. The profits derived from their monopoly let them seek dominance over local outpatient services, and then physician services. As time went on, hospital resources were used to acquire control or ownership of competing outpatient services offered by private practices, such as ambulatory out-patient surgery centers.

Hospitals aim to provide the broadest range of services possible to attract their true customers —physicians. Doctors are the ones who generate patient admissions and referrals for care services. Hospitals work to garner patient revenue from independent physicians. They prefer to employ physicians to capture all revenue from patient services

Profits became necessary for hospitals to finance expanding the range and sophistication of their services. Hospital departments became profit centers. Hospitals wanted fewer loss centers, if any. Those services failing to increase profit margins (or "surpluses" for nonprofit hospitals) were reduced in the budget, eliminated, or contracted out; like anesthesiology.

Margins more than actual community needs began driving the services hospitals offer. As more than one hospital administrator has justified, "There is no mission without a margin."

To deal with competition and declining demands for inpatient capacity, hospitals merged with other hospitals and other sectors of care delivery, like urgent care and out-patient surgery. In this way, a

> Hospitals aim to provide the broadest range of services possible to attract their true customers — physicians. Doctors are the ones who generate patient admissions and referrals for care services.

"healthcare system" was created that not only dominates delivery of care but exploits it economically. Hospitals grew at the expense of the very communities that the hospitals' founders had pledged to serve as the institution's mission, its reason to exist.

Hospitals are compensated for the services provided. The more distinct services are delivered by the hospital system, the greater the revenue. Hospitals today are paid for services by self-pay patients, by insurance companies, and by Medicare and Medicaid. Hospitals are paid more for both Medicare and Medicaid services than these government programs pay to the independent providers.

Hospitals grew at the expense of communities their founders pledged to serve.

Commercial insurance plans negotiate hospital care payments. A monopoly or oligarchy hospital system negotiates from a position of strength in the local geographic area. Pay the demanded rates, the insurers are told, or else don't do business with our local healthcare system and all our patients.

Press releases for nearly every merger promise big cost savings. Blah, blah, blah. Any "savings" achieved by mergers are not accruing to the economic benefit of the community nor the patients.

The Nicholas C. Petris Center at the University of California studied the 25 metropolitan regions in the USA with the highest rates of hospital consolidation between 2010 and 2013. Following a consolidation, the average price of all hospital stays in each locale increased between 11 percent and 54 percent. They also reported increases beyond 25 percent from 2012 to 2014. According to Petris Center director Richard Scheffler, prices rose even more when large hospital systems acquired doctors' groups.

Not every hospital can dominate and exploit its local market. Hospitals can expand their profit margins by negotiating increased reimbursement rates from commercial insurance companies, and by generating a good volume of commercially insured patients. Medicare and Medicaid rates are largely regulated, and rarely profitable. Higher insurance payments to hospitals get passed on to patients as higher service charges, leading to higher insurance premiums.

Hospital administrators see their role as enhancing the economics of their employer. The impact on the community they service be damned. Hospital benefit comes before community benefit.

For local residents with job health coverage, higher group health insurance premiums mean higher payroll deductions when employers pass on their higher costs. As the employers lower the budget impact of insurance premium increases, employees face higher co-pays, higher deductibles, and reductions in coverage.

Adverse impacts on local residents aren't a consideration or concern of hospitals putting self-interest above community service. The pandemic exposed where this was happening.

Downstream Revenues

Hospital systems dominating local health care delivery look to feed their economic interests by capturing downstream revenues — the revenue from care rendered before and after hospitalization. In the same way that Disney World may seek to capture every vacation dollar spent in Orlando by expanding their range of offerings, so too do hospitals seek to capture every healthcare dollar spent in their service areas. Unlike Disney, local hospitals serving local residents run little risk of people vacationing elsewhere.

Profit margins are good. Health insurance companies in 2017 yielded margins between 4.0 and 5.25 percent, reports *Investopedia*. Hospital margins are better. The American Hospital Association's

TrendWatch reported that 23 percent of hospitals show negative margins, but hospitals overall saw 6.4 percent operating margins. The Wisconsin not-for-profit Gundersen Lutheran Medical Center in La Crosse had a pre-Covid annual surplus of $302 million.

Hospital systems often use profit margins from their "medical mission to serve" for growing bigger and dominating more.

Health insurance companies, by law, must spend a percentage of premium revenues on healthcare services or else refund policy holders. Hospitals have no such obligation to use their profits for reducing their charges, or for expanding charity care, or for community betterment. And few do.

Profits instead go toward acquiring more and more hospitals and other medical providers, like physician group practices and urgent care facilities. Healthcare facility mergers and acquisitions tallied 115 transactions in 2017, reported *RevCycle Intelligence*, and that tally increased 11 percent in 2018.

Venture Capitalism

Hospitals now are entering the venture capital business. Indeed, hospitals are a new source of financing for new ideas and businesses. *Forbes* reported that in the first half of 2017, more than $6 billion of hospital money financed startup business ventures.

Hospital systems are creating their own venture capital arms to invest in new businesses, risking mission-driven revenues for future potential economic gains. Most startup ventures fail. The adventure is perilous to a hospital's economic stability. *Becker Hospital Review* in 2019 identified three such investment funds: Ascension Ventures ($800 million), Providence Ventures ($300 million) and United Point Health Ventures ($100 million). Funds generated by VC operations, in theory, could help cover the costs of providing care services for the sick and injured in local communities.

One area of investment is going head-to-head with the insurance companies. Hospital systems know healthcare best, after all, so they figure, "Why not cut out the middleman and create our own health plans? Why not capture insurance margins as our own?"

The reality is different than expected. A 2017 Allan Baumgarten study funded by the Robert Wood Johnson Foundation found that only four of 42 hospital plans were profitable in 2015. Several reported big losses, and five went out of business.

> Hospital systems know healthcare best, after all, so they figure, 'Why not cut out the middleman and create our own health plans?'

Becker's Hospital CFO Report noted that Northwell, based in Long Island, absorbed significant losses from their health insurance startup, CareConnect. Losses on a second insurance plan Northwell owned pushed the company into the red by $36.2 million during the first quarter of 2017, which does not include the loss of all capital in CareConnect.

Premier Health in Ohio, said *Dayton Daily News,* shuttered its insurance plans after a three-year effort with losses of $40 million. Unable to find a buyer, their return on investment was zero.

Some hospital systems are still pushing ahead with their health insurance ventures, plowing in hospital revenues to fund deficits. Other systems are pulling the plug, divesting themselves of losers, as did Catholic Health Initiatives in Englewood, Colorado, and Tenet Healthcare in Dallas. Such economic losses reduce the resources for providing direct health services, especially charity care.

I will not say if these investment strategies are good or bad. I'll raise this question: Should hospital systems be able to increase their charges to private and government payers, and increase costs to the patients, to invest their resources in risky business ventures?

Private business hopes for a high return on investment (ROI), no guarantees. If a venture fails, the hit is taken by the investors, the shareholders. However, a not-for-profit hospital system has no such shareholders. A for-profit-hospital is playing with funds generated by increasing costs to the communities they serve under protected government licenses. Investment losses, if large enough, endanger a hospital's critical medical services.

> Must a community bail out their local hospital because of its appetite for investing in new ventures?

So, I ask: Must a community bail out their local hospital because of its appetite for investing in new ventures? AInd then I ask: Should higher health costs, plus higher premiums, plus higher taxes for Medicare and Medicaid, fund any protected monopoly's attempts to expand its domination over where our medical dollars get spent for personal health care?

Regardless of how hospital systems use their fiscal resources, the public is expected to pick up added operating costs. This includes costs for marketing. Hospital systems invest their revenues in self-aggrandizement — advertising. *FierceHealthcare* estimated that U.S. hospitals spent $10 billion on advertising in 2017 — growing by 1.8 percent every year, projected at $11.5 billion in hospital advertising by 2021. These billions are paid from the care charges demanded of patients directly or through their insurance premiums.

HealthLeaders Magazine has defended marketing expenditures, saying, "Hospitals need to advertise to maintain or enhance revenue flow. Even nonprofit hospitals need to market to insured patients and promote high-grossing service lines, so that they are able to continue to care for the uninsured." No mission without a margin.

Physician-Patient Relationships

The physician-patient relationship is a unique business model. A physician is expected to provide medical knowledge with a high degree of compassion, what the vast majority of physicians do. This poses a challenge for business viability.

A compassionate connection with patients induces independent physicians to write off unpaid bill balances, putting their practices at risk. Employed physicians' compassion for patients is the same, but they have removed themselves from business operations, yet their institutions pay them to maximize revenue. Employed physicians traded independence for a more secure income.

Independent local physicians must sustain their practice as a business, compensating their staff well enough to retain them, yet still derive a decent income themselves, so they can be there for their patients. This difficult, sometimes impossible challenge is why the number of independent physicians is diminishing.

Independent physicians participate in insurance plans to support their patients. Physicians can't get rich on shrinking insurance reimbursements. Their participation lets patients obtain the maximum coverage possible with fewer dollars coming from patients' pockets. Plan participation builds physician-patient relationships by limiting fiscal pressures on their relationships, but participation means less income for physician and subtly strains patient relations.

Lawrence Casalino, MD, PhD., Weill Cornell Medical College, studied physician's practices and found their total cost for dealing with insurance plans was $31 billion annually — 6.9 percent of all U.S. expenditures for physician and clinical services. For patients with limited insurance, or no plan coverage, considerably more time is spent on patient-physician financial arrangements.

The Commonwealth Fund found physicians spent three weeks a year interacting with insurance plans. Nursing staff spent 23 weeks per year per physician. Clerical staff spent 44 weeks. This time could be better spent delivering care, building physician-patient relationships. The staff resources consumed by insurance administration adds nothing to improving care delivery, access or quality.

Patients' total out-of-pocket charges rose from $295 billion in 2008 to $405 billion in 2020.

Fixed care reimbursements, limited sources of payments and increasing expenses has largely eliminated cost-shifting for today's independent physicians. Employed physicians' costs are subsidized by hospitals for referring patients to costlier ancillary services. The independent physician has less options, and little help with the cost of that patient relationship.

For those with health insurance, the patient-physician financial relationship is undergoing a major change. Low co-pays and limited deductibles are fast disappearing. TransUnion Healthcare has reported that patients' average out-of-pocket costs increased 11 percent in 2017, rising to $1,813. About 39 percent of patient visits to physicians incur out-of-pocket costs from $500 to $1,000.

Modern Healthcare reported that out-of-pocket costs increased 14 percent in 2018. The Economic Policy Institute reported that the patient financial responsibility for insured individuals increased 58 percent between 2006 and 2016. Statista reports that patients' total out-of-pocket charges rose from $295.8 billion in 2008 to $405.1 billion in 2020. Collecting on these bills strains the patient-physician relationship and reduces a private medical practice's viability.

For context, the U.S. Bureau of Labor Statistics reported average hourly earnings increased 1 percent annually before the pandemic. It's too much in flux for certainty beyond saying that healthcare cost increases are outstripping increases in personal earnings.

Employed Physicians

Hospital systems grow by adding physicians as employees. Why is that? Isn't more staff more expensive?

About 80 percent of U.S. healthcare spending results from decisions made by physicians. If you control or influence that care decision, you control a significant amount of revenue. Employee physicians yield a regular flow of patients referred to ancillary services owned by the system. System-owned services are paid more than independently owned services, so boosting patient volume assures the system's overall costs for health care will rise.

Laboratory Economics reported that a UnitedHealthcare in-network hospital lab in New York charged 23 times more than did a local LabCorp for the same tests ($384 versus $16.25).

Medical Economics also reported that Medicare paid $188 for a level II EKG without contrast to an independent physician. The same EKG in a hospital's outpatient setting cost 140 percent more ($452.89) when charged by the employed physician.

Costs from hospital-employed physicians are draining the financial stability of Medicare. *Modern Healthcare Magazine* in November 2017 ran an analysis of U.S. costs for four procedures at hospital outpatient services compared with independent locations. Employed physicians generated 27 percent more Medicare costs

($3.1 billion) than did independent physicians. The employed physicians were seven times more likely to provide services in a more costly hospital outpatient setting.

Employed physicians, motivated by convenience and loyalty, are likely to refer patients to their employers' ancillary services, such as imaging. A *New York Times* story about mergers quoted a healthcare worker's online comment, "Each month MDs receive a 'report card' that measures the 'leakage,' i.e., services ordered by the MD that are done by a non-affiliated provider." If a patient chooses to have an MRI or cardiac consultation done at an independent facility, "the staff in the physician's office must document why the service was not directed to an affiliated provider."

> Employed physicians, motivated by convenience and loyalty, are likely to refer patients to their employers' ancillary services.

My own explanation is that conscious patients knew enough about their insurance coverage, knew what would be their out-of-pocket costs, and for quality of care insisted upon a referral to an independent provider.

An Empire Blue Cross executive said the cost of care provided by an employed physician is 20 to 40 percent higher than the cost of that same care by a physician in independent practice.

Hospitals' employment of physicians is increasing dramatically. In the year ending July 2016, hospitals acquired 5,000 physician practices, reported *Healthcare Dive*. Separately, *FierceHealthcare* reported that hospital-owned practices increased 100 percent in the four years ending in 2016. Nationally, 38 percent of all physician practices are now hospital-owned.

The fast pace of consolidating physicians under employment contracts is even higher today. *Becker's ASC Review* in July 2021 reported that 70 percent of all U.S. physicians are now employed by hospitals or corporations. Thirty percent are independent.

Independent Physicians

Local independent physicians are fighting a rearguard action.

Independent physician practices may be a vanishing breed, but individual physicians in small practices are the providers of choice for most of the frequent medical care people receive.

Independent physicians face a greater economic burden than those employed by hospital-owned practices, and they have far less flexibility in revenue generation. Regulations don't favor them in attempting financial creativity and "revenue maximization."

At the same time, health insurance plans focus their economic considerations on the dominant hospitals and their employed staff physicians. Insurers try to shift the burden of their aggregate cost increases onto the backs of the independents, who seldom have the market leverage to withstand the pressure.

The 2018 *Survey of America's Physicians* revealed an evolving medical profession struggling with burnout and low morale. Only 31 percent of physicians identified as independent practice owners or partners, down from 33 percent in 2016, itself down from 48.5 percent in 2012. Independent physicians are a shrinking minority.

Most independent practices are in the medical specialties. These physicians directly affect the lives and wellbeing of their patients. They include the family practitioners, obstetricians/gynecologists, internists, oncologists, and orthopedic surgeons, to name few of the many medical specialists who rely on good reputations.

Beyond their responsibilities for the delivery of medical care, the independent physicians must endure the pressures and concerns of any small business, like staff payroll. A Kaiser Foundation report, "Professional Active Physicians," estimates small practices employ more than five million people in the USA. Each physician pays for a median of six employees.

> Beyond their responsibilities for the delivery of medical care, the independent physicians must endure the pressures and concerns of any small business.

Independent physicians' sole source of revenue is the sale and delivery of professional expertise and specialized knowledge, generally sold in units of time. Time is their finite resource. Physicians who spend extra time with their grateful patients, in fiscal reality, put their practices at risk.

A good video, "The Vanishing Oath," narrated by Ryan Flesher, MD, gives us a clear sense of the financial realities of the "average" physician. The average compensation for independent physicians in the USA is about three times the national average for household income. However, when you factor in overhead and working hours, physicians' take-home pay averages less than $28 an hour. It's above minimum wage of $15 an hour, but not by much.

The average charge for more than 200 million visits paid by Medicare in 2012 was just $57, less than a plumber charges to fix a broken toilet, says Nancy Nielsen, MD, PhD. a past president of the American Medical Association, as reported by *MedPage Today*.

Compensation of employed physicians is similar to those in independent practices. *Physician Practice* in 2018 reported that 69.5 percent of physicians who own their practice bring home more than $200,000 in annual compensation. That's slightly less income than the 75.3 percent for employed physicians. If income is similar for employed and private physicians, what's the difference?

What's different is that physicians in private practice carry the weight of operating an increasingly complex business without the staff support of hospital practices. Independents are responsible for 100 percent of their net income, based on their own labor.

A fact of physician life is the burden of debt from a medical education. The National Center for Education Statistics estimates medical students graduating in 2019 had $232,300 in debt. This debt affects where they choose to practice, especially whether they are independent or employed.

In communities where a population is economically challenged, private practice physicians are in short supply. Practice costs cannot be met through a high volume of low-paying Medicaid patients, not without the quality of their care suffering. Therefore, physicians tend to congregate in the high-income suburbs or upscale urban neighborhoods. Where and how such physicians practice medicine becomes more about their lifestyle and economics than meeting a community's health care needs.

Affordable Care Act Impacts

The Affordable Care Act increased health insurance coverage while increasing the economic burden of care. The ACA added to the intensity of the patient-physician financial exchange.

The debate over "health reform" turned into a plan for getting all Americans covered by health insurance. We talked a lot about the cost of coverage but little about what it cost to obtain that coverage.

Coverage did not cover everything from the first dollar onward. To get the broad coverage of the mandated benefit plans, patients had to accept higher deductibles. In theory, this would "engage" patients in seeing that care is not free, so they're judicious in its use.

In reality, cancer patients would be happy never to need care services, but they have no choice. High deductibles sting the necessary users of medical care as well as the unnecessary users.

There was much talk about premium costs, how there would be tax credits for businesses to offer coverage. There'd be subsidies to provide for individuals to buy coverage, and the "essential benefits" that had to be included. What it all would cost patients to access care received short shrift in the conversations.

With ACA subsidies cushioning the economics of purchasing coverage with such essential benefits as "free" preventive care and coverage for preexisting conditions, the sticker shock of deductibles only hits us when there's an illness or injury. That's when the out-of-pocket costs can decide whether people actually choose to seek the care needed for themselves or their family members.

Covid Impacts

The Covid-19 pandemic laid bare the deficiencies of healthcare financing and service delivery systems.

In the 2020 Covid wave and the 2021 surge of the virulent Delta variant, hospitals have had to make provisions for expected Covid patients, even if they did not materialize. Hospitals have curtailed elective services, their main sources of revenue from both inpatient and outpatient. At the same time, patients, and potential patients have curtailed their regular, urgent and even emergency use of hospital facilities, further eliminating hospital revenues. Hospital utilization was "feast or famine." Facilities have been overwhelmed by Covid or else sitting empty.

Meanwhile, operating costs continued, skyrocketing from price competition for scarce supplies and competent staffing. Hospitals responded by cutting staff. Some decided, for instance, they don't need to staff surgical services at prior levels. Surgical procedures dropped 53 percent from January 2018 to June 2020. Cardiovascular Research Foundation in February 2021 reported that elective cases dropped by 65 percent, and non-elective cases dropped 40 percent. Similar staffing cuts occurred for every hospital service not engaged in treating Covid cases.

Hospital revenues are tied to serving the sick and injured with a mixture of both profitable and non-profitable patients. *Becker's Hospital CFO Report* documented in early 2020 that 879 hospitals were at risk of closure, most of them rural facilities.

It's a fallacy to expect our community hospitals to be available in times of need, yet they survive only from earnings when needed. It's like expecting police and fire departments to be always ready, yet paying them only when they respond to crime or a fire.

> It's a fallacy to expect our community hospitals to be fully available in times of need, yet they survive only from earnings when needed.

The fate of physicians employed by hospitals during Covid largely follows the fate of their employers. Physicians active in providing Covid care work exhausting hours, for which they get more income. Independent physicians specializing in care with reduced demand, when the patent volume drops, face reduced hours, or even layoffs, both for themselves and their supporting staff.

For physicians in private practice, their fate has been left to their ingenuity. The same goes for non-physician care givers, such as behavioral health counselors. They've had to innovate.

With Covid-cautious patients afraid of going to an office, tele-medicine became the new revenue channel. This new "source of treatment" provides some income. When Medicare, Medicaid and private insurance provide payment for telemedicine, those rates do not match the reimbursements for office visits. Telemedicine has proven popular with patients, but reimbursements are expected to end as the pandemic relents.

In response to the revenues losses from Covid, independent physicians increasingly are looking for the shelter of employment by a hospital or a physicians group. Other physicians are choosing retirement earlier than planned. The Physician's Foundation in July 2020 reported that 59 percent of the physicians surveyed said the pandemic resulted in an overall reduction of independent physicians in their communities. The pandemic may herald the long-expected demise of the small medical practice.

Healthcare Values vs. Costs

Probably the greatest challenge facing physicians is the value Americans place on healthcare compared with its costs. In general, healthcare costs are perceived as too high and the quality as too low. Patient satisfaction and customer service levels? Even lower.

Physicians are easy targets for efforts to control costs. They're on the receiving end of bureaucratic rules set to "improve quality." Employed physicians have hospital resources to lessen bureaucratic burdens. Independent physicians are on their own.

Unlike other small businesses, physicians' income is largely out of their control. Businesses adapt prices to cost and competition. Physicians' reimbursements are now dictated to them.

Physicians agree to accept the fixed rates from private health plans in exchange for plan participation. Medicare pays fixed rates to physicians for seniors, the largest consumers of medical care services. Each state sets its own fixed Medicaid rates.

Physicians in a hospital practice benefit from their monopolistic hospital assuring its paid higher rates by insurance, but independent physicians have little leverage to negotiate with commercial health plans. For private practices, insurance plan participation is a take-it-or-leave-it proposition.

Commercial plans foolishly give short-shrift to independent providers. Satisfying the demands of monopolistic medical care systems, health insurers are driving independent physicians into hospital employment. The result is higher costs for physician fees and all the services they provide.

> Satisfying the demands of monopolistic care systems, health insurers are driving independent physicians into hospital employment.

Unique in medicine is that physicians' compensation is tied to a service or procedure, regardless of a given physicians' experience to improve the quality and efficiency of the care being delivered. A surgeon removing an appendix is paid the same amount regardless of whether she or he is a veteran of thousands of appendectomies or a recent graduate with the ink still wet on the medical license.

While patients naturally want the most experienced physician, is the physician's experience being valued or respected by insurance and government plans? I think not.

Despite the perennial cry, "The sky is falling!" physicians are not dropping out of Medicare in droves. The Centers for Medicare & Medicaid Service (CMS) say that 90 percent of practicing physicians accept Medicare patients. *Kaiser Health News* says that 69 percent participate with Medicaid. These numbers are holding steady.

Physician participation in the commercial insurance plans is increasing while benefit coverage is shrinking. It's being eliminated for health services provided by physicians who do not participate with commercial plans. For many physicians, especially in private practice, plan participations is about taking off their patients the economic burden for needed care. It's far less about maximizing the physicians' income.

> Patients are learning to match their care to their coverage, avoiding higher out-of-pocket costs.

As deductibles have risen, independent physicians, for the survival of their private practices, increasingly must play the role of bill collector with their patients.

Meanwhile, more patients are learning to match their care to their coverage, avoiding higher out-of-pocket costs, avoiding the big bills for care provided by out-of-network physicians.

Insurance companies have been less than generous in sharing their increasing premium revenue over the last ten to twelve years. *MD Magazine* reports on the discouraging slide of payment rates to physicians since 2001, saying they have declined or remained flat almost every year, a trend likely to continue.

Payments to physicians from commercial plans are running less than Medicare. Between 2006 and 2013, payments dropped about

43 percent. *Medscape* calculated that payment for the most common types of office visit is 39 percent less than what Medicare pays.

Patients need to understand that their physicians, all physicians, sell their time. Time remains a limited resource.

For independent physicians in private practice, insurance reimbursements are falling behind their costs to stay in business. From 2002 to 2012, Medicare fee-for-service (FFS) rates increased nine percent, while the cost of operating a practice, measured by the Medicare Economic Index (MEI), increased 27 percent, reported the Medicare Payment Advisory Commission (MedPac). The MEI includes everything from physician and staff compensation to rent, exam tables, postage, and computers. During that very same period, the overall inflation rate was 33 percent — a net loss.

The Physician's Dilemma

High deductibles and co-pays become "account receivables" for physicians and then medical debt for patients. Affordability is not academic for physicians in their practice. For them, it's a tangible challenge to their financial survival as well as their ability to provide proper care for their patients.

Given fixed or declining care reimbursements from insurance, given increased operating costs, our independent physicians face a conflict between the doctor-patient relationship and the patient-doctor financial exchange.

Physician-patient relationships give physicians more knowledge of patients' situations than usual business transactions. An intimate knowledge of patients' fiscal circumstances creates tension.

The patients who need the most physician or other medical care and services often have the most economic issues, perhaps caused by illness or injury, or as a consequence of the stress. These patients frequently cannot work, or they're restricted in their ability to work, requiring time and attention by family members, who may decide caregiving takes priority over producing income.

The physician's dilemma: With limited time to care for patients and earn revenue, with fixed reimbursements limiting their income, how can they balance the economic needs of their practice with a compassionate response to each patient's situation?

Head vs. Heart

Physicians in private practice must generate sufficient income to cover expenses of their practice and support their own families. When payments from insurance are insufficient, due to poor coverage or limitations on coverage, the patient is fully responsible.

Independent physicians know in their heads that any heart-guided write-offs of patients' debt can spell financial ruin for their practice. This emotional and ethical struggle between the head and the heart is seldom faced in other businesses.

"Hard core" bill collections against patients, who likely have medical and financial problems, are contrary to most physicians' personal values and sentiments. Physicians add to patients' debt load, not out of desire, but out of economic necessity.

In their hearts, physicians feel an impulse to forgive patient debt. With their head, they know that they cannot absorb the fiscal loss, nor can they risk sanctions from insurance carriers.

What should independent physicians do? What would you do?

The easiest course is removing oneself from the business of medicine to be an employee of a large organization or institution. Free yourself to practice medicine. Be unburdened from business administration, billing and collections. Turn over those distasteful tasks to your institution. However, doing so means your patients will not be buffered by your compassion, as billing for services you provide go into a system designed to maximize revenue.

The billing and collections on behalf of hospital-employed physicians reflect the processes and programs of that institution. While every hospital has a policy for charity care, there is little outreach to ensure wise use of the funds. In fact, since the advent of the ACA, with more people being covered under state Medicaid, says the Advisory Board, the use of charity funds by hospitals has fallen to less than two percent of their operating costs.

> In their hearts, physicians feel an impulse to forgive patient debt. In their heads, they know that they cannot absorb the fiscal loss.

Under the ACA, as insurance plan deductibles rise, the middle class suffers a gigantic increase in medical debt. This demographic mostly has insurance, but they do not think of seeking charity care from local hospitals, especially at the time of service. Or, they may think of it, but feel too ashamed to ask, Accepting charity is a stigma, and they're proud, so proud they go into debt.

Sadly, if heavily burdened people in the middle class would ask for charity care or sliding scale rates, few would qualify. They're too rich for assistance, yet too poor to afford the bill.

Only when the bills arrive do the gaps in plan coverage become evident. Only then are tangible burdens of medical debt understood. By then, the patient is out of the hospital. The sign in Admissions, inviting inquiries for charity care, is long forgotten. Hospitals do not go out of their way to promote or offer charity care to patients. A bill or demand for payment for care services seldom offers any relief by contacting the hospital to make arrangements.

Independent practices that sell their medical debt are few and far between, and fewer ask an agency to pursue collections in court or report their bad debt to credit bureaus. However, hospital-owned medical practices, following a hospital's practices, regularly file legal action and regularly report bad accounts to credit bureaus.

Another twist causing medical debt is that hospitals which do provide charity care, if barely, could seek better compensation rates, or community support to fund charity care. However, not-for-profit hospitals instead focus on raising funds to provide new services that increase revenue, which then increases medical debt.

Independent physicians lack the institutional or community support for a heartfelt campaign to end the medical debt of hardship patients. There is no support for any increase in their rates, so they cannot afford to provide charity care, but many do.

Absorbing the medical debt of patients who need care but can't afford it, bluntly, is another reason to abandon private independent medical practice to join a hospital-owned practice. That choice for personal survival by independent physicians results in higher costs for health care, increasing medical debt in a community.

Independent physicians seek to provide for their patients, their employees, their own families, and their communities. They choose mission over margin, choose heart over head, yet they do so at their fiscal peril, and they alone are expected to pick up the tab.

Hospital systems tend to choose profit margin over missions of service, put mission in service to margin. Despite all the compassion of hospital leaders, institutional needs compel them to choose head over heart, to exploit every opportunity for market dominance. Our society is expected to pick up the tab. Is this sensible?

CHAPTER 7

Fanciful Healthcare Financing

Robert E. Goff

I believe insurance is the wrong way to finance the healthcare needs of Americans. Covid's ruinous impact on the current healthcare financing structure only supports my conviction.

I come to this belief honestly, only after decades in healthcare management at the highest levels.

To understand why I say insurance is the wrong way to finance the healthcare needs of Americans, I offer here a brief education on how insurance actually works, in practical terms, and a brief history of health insurance, tracing back to war and tax policies.

Insurance is a financial device to absorb economic consequences of rare events. Insurance provides money to policyholder to restore physical damage from a covered incident. Property insurance works well for homes and autos, so I'll use that as an example.

The financing of insurance is relatively simple. A company offers to provide coverage for these rare events. The risk is spread over all the policyholders, allowing each to pay a small amount on a regular basis to cover costs of any policyholder should that rare event occur. Policyholders, essentially, fund one another's losses. The insurance company holds on to the funds not paid out, keeping a portion for administration and profit.

To avoid those rare events that must be covered, or to mitigate the impact, insurance companies promote safety. Policyholders are encouraged to conduct themselves in ways that reduce risk.

Insurance companies offer policyholders financial incentives to reduce claims, such as discounts for taking a safe driving class or for vehicle safety features. Likewise, they offer premium discounts for home security features, such as smoke and burglar alarms.

Policyholders assume part of the fiscal impact from rare events through deductibles. Homeowners or vehicle owners who become "high utilizers" of insurance coverage, or potentially high utilizers — like living in a flood plain or having a poor driving record — may find insurance coverage unaffordable or unavailable.

Lastly, homeowners' insurance policies and auto policies contain "caps" or limits on their coverage. Because homes and automobiles have market values, which can be established, insurance companies do not want to overpay in reimbursing the cost of damages. Limiting the liability of the insurance carrier is accepted in the law.

Healthcare Insurance Business Model

Applying property insurance concepts to financing healthcare, in my view, is simply wrongheaded. An individual's need for health services is not a rare event. It's expected, perhaps predictable. Illness and injury are commonplace. For example, few mothers give birth today without any intervention by medical services, and few deaths occur without some medical interventions.

Health care occurs lifelong. A childhood rite of passage is all the preventive care like immunizations and checkups. In adolescence,

HPV vaccinations can protect against certain cancers. For young women, a Pap test for cervical cancer is an annual rite, like mammograms for older women. As men mature, PSA prostate cancer screening is routine. Colonoscopies after age 50 are advised for all. Routine annual physicals are chances to screen for basic health issues, like diabetes or high blood pressure. Good health insurance covers usual and expected events in life to assure good health.

The business model of covering the rare events, as expected for other forms of insurance, does not fit health insurance. Unlike with a vehicle or a house, we do not place a market value on human life.

> Applying property insurance concepts to financing healthcare is simply wrongheaded.

As you age, your statistical chances increase of developing one or more chronic health conditions. As medical science improves, your chances increase for living through an acute illness like appendicitis or pneumonia. Cancer treatments have made that killer survivable for more than ever. Cardiac surgery is considered safe and routine. Americans today live through the episodic health crises that in past generations would have ended life. By living longer, we live long enough to develop and live with chronic illnesses. We expect health insurance to cover it all from cradle to grave.

Yes, unfortunate catastrophic and rare illnesses do occur, but 45 percent of the population, 133 million Americans, have at least one chronic disease, reported the Partnership to Fight Chronic Disease, and 26 percent are living with two or more conditions. The Clearing House Advisory Committee calculated chronic diseases account for three of every four dollars of health care spending. Total health care spending in 2019 surpassed $3.6 trillion, according to a report from Fitch Solutions Macro Research. Close to 99 percent of Medicare and 83 percent of the Medicaid expenditures are for chronic care. The older we get, the more costly is our care.

The healthcare insurance model is designed to provide financial assistance for rare events, but instead it is expected to fund health care needs that are no longer rare, to fund needs that are not only predictable but expected. Such financing is fanciful.

High Health Insurance Premiums

The rising cost of health insurance premiums gets bashed in the healthcare debate. Critics vilify insurance company profits, big CEO salaries and wasteful administration. Often forgotten is the fact that premiums largely reflect the hard costs of medical services, the *unit cost* of each service, and the volume of services utilized.

Now add in the cost to operate an insurance company, including claims payments, marketing, and efforts to influence utilization of health services, plus a margin for profitability.

Health insurance premiums follow a simple equation:

Medical costs + administrative costs + profits = premiums.

The National Association of Insurance Commissioners (NAIC) in 2018 reported basic industry profitability at 3.3 percent, which is far below the public perception that profits are in the range of 10 to 25 percent. (The average profit margin for an S&P 500 company in the last quarter of 2020 was 10.3. percent, dropping after a year of pandemic from the 10.9 percent five-year average.

To hold down premiums, health insurance companies mimic the devices of property and casualty insurance to mitigate their risk of claims. They encouraging people to adopt healthy habits with insurance "motivators," but these are undercut by deductibles.

Prior to the Affordable Care Act (Obamacare), health insurance companies often reduced their risks of medical claims by excluding coverage for preexisting conditions. They imposed waiting periods before coverage began. They excluded individuals and small groups, requiring enough policyholders to spread the risks. The business case set coverage limits.

No health insurance company can survive or provide coverage for anyone if the only people who buy policies are those who require medical care. Similarly, no auto insurance company can survive selling policies only to people with poor driving records who have had lots of accidents.

Medical costs
+ admin costs
+ profit margin
= premiums.

Such fiscal pragmatism is the basis of the ACA requirement that everyone must purchase health coverage. The "individual mandate" served two purposes. First, spread the costs of care across the broadest number of insurance premium payers, in theory, reducing each one's contribution. Second, assure everyone was covered.

Health insurance emulates property insurance on deductibles. By setting a personal financial responsibility requirement before care, it limits or caps outlay before care services are covered. Just like caps on coverage for homeowners and auto insurance, lifetime health insurance caps of $250,000, $500,000 and even $1 million were not uncommon. The ACA banned lifetime caps and limits. Big change! Insurance companies now must pay all valid claims without any end in sight. They mitigate the fiscal stress by increasing premiums.

Before the ACA, deductibles were a disincentive to preventative care. The ACA requires insurance companies to cover preventive care services without a copayment or coinsurance, even if a patient has not met the annual deductible. The preventive care rule requires an additional outlay by health insurance companies.

The individual mandate was effectively nullified by pulling its teeth with courts ruling against fines for not having insurance. This loss means the risk of medical cost cannot be spread out among the nearly everyone. Since the basis of insurance financing is spreading out the risk and cost, premiums by necessity will rise.

You may or may not agree with the individual mandate, but in practical terms, its repeal has added to the reasons health insurance companies are raising policy premiums to stay in business.

Insurance Funds Medical Advances

Health insurance, for all its criticisms, should be complimented for dramatic improvements in the sophistication of health services. All those dollars paid by insurance companies — plus by Medicare for the aged and Medicaid for the poor — become income for health care providers. Health insurance allowed medical caregivers to end their dependency on charity, replacing pleas for donations with a dependable source of funding. Another big change.

Reliable funding from health insurance has been a stimulus for expanding medical research and transferring research into practical use. Reliable funding allows medical device makers, pharmaceutical companies, and research hospitals to develop new lifesaving medical technologies that otherwise would lack funding.

Consider the 1972 expansion of Medicare to cover people with End State Renal Disease (ESRD), kidney failure. Before then, there was limited investment in dialysis machines and services, mostly at academic medical centers. Patient access to limited life-continuing treatments was decided by committees.

Access to funds means access to care. From Medicare expansion, more patients with ESRD began to survive. The U.S. Renal Data

System in 2016 reported close to 350,000 people having a primary diagnosis of renal failure. In 2013, Medicare reported its costs for treating patients with chronic kidney disease (CKD) surpassed $50 billion, representing 20 percent of all Medicare spending for those over 65 years old.

Patients surviving renal failure live with other chronic diseases. Seventy percent of Medicare spending for CKD patients over age 65 had diabetes, congestive heart failure, or both. Between 2010 and 2013, Medicare patients with chronic conditions accounted for $8 billion of the $9 billion total growth in Medicare spending.

Health insurance has funded medical advancements, yet with a significant advance in costs.

Early History of Health Insurance

If medical care costs are now routine, expected and predictable, then a financing model designed for rare events is not a model for successfully financing healthcare, nor for improving the health status of Americans. How did we land in our current circumstances?

The USA is the only country in the industrialized world without a national health care plan, some form of nationalized coverage. Is there some evil cabal pulling the strings? Is there a series of unfortunate decisions or non-decisions, coupled with ideology?

In early America, if you got sick, you lived or died. Medical care, if available, cost little.

How we got into this sorry situation, historically, is a lack of national leadership, coupled with competing ideas or philosophies on personal responsibility versus collective responsibility.

In early America, individual health was an individual and family responsibility. Birth was at home, often attended by older women in the community. Preventive care meant, "An apple a day keeps the doctor away." No immunizations. No cancer screening. If you got sick, you lived or died. Medical care, if available, cost little.

As cities grew, people living in close quarters raised concerns of communicable diseases. Port cities made efforts to stop sailors or immigrants carrying diseases. Early hospitals cared for those without families and quarantined with infectious illnesses. For example, tuberculosis ravaged the urban poor in the late 19th and early 20th centuries, leading to TB "sanitarium" hospitals in rural areas.

Immigrants from the old country formed "benevolent" associations to help each other in the new one. Early credit unions and burial societies served religious or ethnic groups. Regular payments by all members funded payments to any member who got ill or injured.

> ## Immigrants from the old country formed associations to help each other in the new one.

Commercial insurance started before the Civil War to cover feared injuries from steamboat or railroad travel. Massachusetts Health Insurance in Boston offered an early group insurance policy in 1847.

Industrial age employers began to pay for the health care of employees and their families. You can't run a factory if the employees are out sick at home. "Company towns" offered company physicians and clinics. Chancellor Otto von Bismarck in 1884 mandated health coverage for all Germans from the very same motive: A strong military requires a healthy population.

Modern health insurance got its start in the Great Depression. With fewer patients able to pay, and those with jobs facing hardship if they became ill, hospitals began to offer insurance for the costs of hospital care. A network of community hospital insurance companies united as the Blue Cross, based on a 1920s offer by Baylor University Hospital to Dallas public school teachers. Baylor provided hospital services to teachers at 50 cents a month. Physician's charges were not covered, so physicians united to form the national Blue Shield in 1939. The Blue Cross and Blue Shield federations merged in 1982, becoming among the five biggest health insurors today.

> # Modern health insurance got its start in the Great Depression.

After the Depression gave rise to modern health insurance, World War II spawned employer-sponsored health insurance.

Military conscription created labor shortages, yet factories had to increase their labor force to meet wartime production. Government wage controls limited the ability to offer higher wages, so factories turned to fringe benefits for attracting workers. Health benefits, the more generous the better, became a vital recruitment tool.

Employer-sponsored health insurance got a boost in 1943 when the Internal Revenue Service ruled that the cost of health insurance, if provided through an employer, was tax-free to the employee and tax-deductible for the employer. This tax advantage for employer-sponsored health insurance was reconfirmed in 1954.

Nine percent of the population was covered by voluntary private health insurance in 1940, growing to 63 percent by 1953 and then 70 percent in the 1960s, according to an NPR *Planet Money* report. Private health insurance seemed to be working for America.

Advent of Medicare and Medicaid

Two dark clouds hovered over private health insurance from the not-for-profit insurers like Blue Cross and Blue Shield as well as the commercial for-profit companies like Aetna. Poor people not in the workforce, and the those over age 65 aging out of the workforce, were not being covered by health insurance.

Medical care extended people's lives beyond their working years, yet older people were being impoverished by health care costs. The poor and unemployed, relegated to charity care, were squeezed by the costs of medical advances.

Americans do not like the idea of people dying on the street, or seeing their parents (who spent a lifetime working hard) retire into abject poverty brought on by high health care costs. Something had to be done. Congress responded in 1960 with the Kerr-Mills Act to match state funds for patients' bills, but it was not enough.

After wrangling, as a part of President Lyndon Johnson's Great Society, Congress in 1965 enacted Medicare for people over age 65 and Medicaid for the poor.

Medicare's insurance premium is funded in a person's worklife from payroll deductions and employer contributions.

Medicaid is funded by federal taxes, allocated based on state poverty levels, plus state and local taxes. States control Medicaid benefit levels. Local counties control individual enrollments.

Health insurance companies did not oppose Medicaid because poor people were not potential customers. For medical providers, especially for hospitals, Medicaid meant more reliable money than was possible from donations for charity care.

Private physicians were different. Many willingly provided care to poor patients without compensation, so now they could be paid by Medicaid. But bureaucracy intervened in what physicians saw as a moral duty, making it a commercial transaction, shifting the focus from healing to business. Some physicians refused to participate in Medicaid and yet still provided unpaid health care to the poor.

Medicare, in contrast, was initially opposed by the commercial insurance industry. Then logic set in. People work until age 65 and retire in relative health. When their big medical bills roll in, they're on Medicare, not private insurance, so no loss of profits!

The medical community itself was harder to convince.

The medical establishment's enthusiasm was dampened by the potential of big government, any third party, taking a role in patient care, influencing or commanding care activities, impacting the physician-patient relationship. Then they saw Medicare could improve physicians' incomes since patients needing their services now had a reliable funding source. Initially, care services were virtually unconstrained, and payments reflected a high percentage of the customary fees for medical care.

Health insurance companies did not oppose Medicaid because poor people were not potential customers.

Here was the vision: Employer-sponsored health insurance for the workers. Medicare for the elderly. Medicaid for the poor. Gaps in coverage from unemployment were handled by the Consolidated Omnibus Budget Reconciliation Act (COBRA), letting individuals extend their employer-sponsored health insurance up to 18 months, paying the premiums themselves until they found another job.

Virtually everyone was covered. What could go wrong?

What Went Wrong

In theory, all was right with the world. What went wrong was costs emulating New York State's motto, *excelsior*, ever upward.

From a nominal expenditure by employers and taxpayers, health insurance costs grew into expenditures sucking up more and more dollars. The Centers for Disease Control reported health care costs in 1960 were $26 billion, 5.2 percent of the Gross Domestic Product. Costs in 1990 were $725 billion (2.4 percent of GDP). CDC projects healthcare by 2025 at $5 trillion (20 percent of GDP).

Meanwhile, worker's contributions for health insurance benefits reduces their take-home pay, as do the increased Medicare payroll deductions. Medicaid use keeps pushing up federal, state and local taxes. This health insurance model worked until the costs of care drove premiums and tax support past the point of pain.

The gold mine of health insurance financed physicians, hospitals, pharmaceuticals, medical supplies and device manufacturers, the care providers of all types. As new and improved services rushed to meet ever-growing patient needs, costs continued to grow.

Hospitals had to purchase the very latest diagnostic equipment. [Ed. ref. *Arrowsmith* by Sinclair Lewis.] Radiology got a CT scanner, then an MRI. By 2016, the USA had nearly 37 MRI machines for each million people, according to Statista. Canada had nine MRIs for each million people. All of this hiked hospital costs.

The payment model for insured health care services was both simple and inflationary. Policyholders accepted that care services offered were deemed effective and medically necessary, so insurance would cover all costs up to policy limits. The limits were generous as a high percentage of "usual and customary" charges. But the U&C charges then skyrocketed. As long as physicians agreed to accept insurance payments in full, patients willingly or unwittingly played along.

Health insurance paid for it all, virtually without any question. Multiple visits for the same condition, even hospitalization for the convenience of a family, like admitting Mom so children could go on vacation. Effectiveness was not tracked, nor was quality. If some medical error required hospital re-admission, health insurance paid the bill without question. Happy days in healthcare.

As the cost of healthcare rose, so did health insurance premiums, so did Medicare premiums, and so did taxes to support Medicaid. The easy focus was (and to a large degree remains) on consumer costs for health insurance, Medicare, and on what taxpayers pay for Medicaid. The actual culprit is the hard cost of medical services. As costs grew, so did all the schemes and plans to constrain them and pay them.

States stepped in to limit the unit costs for services provided to Medicaid recipients. Medicare set a schedule of its allowable fees. Commercial insurance passed on cost increases to employers, who passed them on to employees as increased payroll deductions.

> This health insurance model worked until the costs of care drove premiums and tax support past the point of pain.

Hospitals in many states came under laws that tried to control the rates they charged. Medicare moved from payments based on length of hospital stay to payments based on diagnosis.

Commercial plans reduced premiums by reducing benefits, such as not covering physician visits unless the patient had an illness (so much for preventive care), increasing co-pays at the time of service, and by tightening underwriting on who they would insure.

Managed Care

The most impactful scheme to "bend the cost curve," to restrain the rate of cost growth, was a model Henry Kaiser developed during construction of the Hoover Dam, later used in the shipyard where Liberty ships were mass-produced during World War II.

The "managed care" model of a *health maintenance organization* (HMO) approached costs, quality and bureaucracy differently.

The original Kaiser model called for the insurer to control the medical delivery system, to manage individuals' care throughout the system, eliminate waste and duplication, monitor quality, and implement treatment plans proven as the most effective for the least cost. The resulting cost to the patient and to the employer could be constrained. This became the Kaiser Permanente Health Plan.

HMOs took off. What began as a movement expected to enroll 20% of the population has become the universal model for delivering care.

The goal of managed care was to serve the long-term interests of patients' health. Offer easy access to primary care physicians, so the patients saw physicians early on in any illness. Early interventions lowered the costs. Benefits were enhanced. The lifetime caps were removed. By owning a full system of hospitals, outpatient services and physicians, HMOs were motivated to provide care in the least costly settings.

The fly in the medicinal ointment? Patients were required to use the HMO's system hospitals and physicians *only*. Corralling

Americans into such a system met with resistance. President Nixon in 1973 signed the Health Maintenance Organization Act (HMO Act). Sen. Edward M. Kennedy was the primary sponsor.

HMOs took off. What began as a movement expected to enroll 20 percent of the population has become the universal model for delivering coverage, not only for employer-sponsored health plans, but also Medicare and Medicaid. HMOs initially were, indeed, able to put the brakes on costs, chiefly care unit costs, as they contracted with medical providers and hospitals at discounted rates.

As physicians had feared with the advent of Medicare, adding a third party into patient-physician relationships altered the nature of the relationship. The HMOs moved beyond controlling unit costs to managing care itself. Sparks began to fly.

Patients did not want to stay restricted to the HMO's network, and they did not like having to get permission to go see a specialist. Medical providers did not want to be told to whom they could refer patients, nor be pressured to use unsure alternatives to traditional treatment plans, such as outpatient care. Horror stories told about patients limited to "in-network" coverage and then getting deficient or timely access to quality care by in-network providers.

Although much went wrong with HMOs, much went right, too. For a period of time, cost increases stabilized. However, the initial HMO strategy could not hold down costs long-term.

Market resentment toward "managed care," by both patients and physicians, doomed the underlying model. Over time, inflationary fee-for-service models returned as the norm, as it is today.

The Affordable Care Act

Health insurance premiums kept on increasing by double digits, two to three times the rate of inflation. Employers balanced the costs by passing along rate increases through higher payroll deductions and fewer wage increases. States grappled with Medicaid costs by cutting fees paid for medical services. Medicare restrained costs by cutting hospital rates and limiting increases in physician fees.

Insurance companies tried to slow cost increases. Individual and small group policies then became unavailable or unaffordable. Small businesses gave up and dropped worker coverage completely.

The Great Recession of 2008 became the great disrupter in health insurance. The ensuing reform, the Affordable Care Act, derisively or proudly called Obamacare, changed health insurance dramatically without changing the basic structure of care delivery.

The concept is simple. Get 100 percent of the U.S. population insured. With everyone insured, every citizen would have coverage, forever removing economics as a barrier to healthcare services. All would be protected from financial devastation for necessary care. The cost of delivering care would be spread over the entire population by mandate, in effect nationalizing the costs for medical care, but *not* the delivery of care. No exclusions

The ACA's big promises were more political than practical.

for preexisting conditions. No lifetime caps. Affordable health insurance no longer would be available only through an employer.

In the ACA vision, hospitals, doctors and other caregivers would no longer carry the bad debt of providing services without payment, passing on to others the costs of uncompensated care. Don't force all people into one plan. Let them choose from among comparable plans in a digital exchange Marketplace. Let them pick a plan based on price, reputation and it's network of hospitals and physicians. Reduce the confusion in plan selection by mandating four benefit packages labeled as Bronze, Silver, Gold, and Platinum.

For those with low income who can't afford a metallic ACA plan, expand Medicaid eligibility to those with incomes up to 132 percent of the Federal Poverty Level (FPL).

For those of modest means, between 133 and 400 percent of the FPL, subsidize their purchase of "approved" metallic plans.

The ACA's big promises were more political than practical. President Obama's vow — "If you like your doctor, you can keep your doctor!" — had a huge asterisk. The ability to keep your doctor depends on whether or not your doctor chooses to participate in a selected ACA-approved plan's network of providers.

For approved plans with standard benefits under metallic labels, they differentiated on price and their network of medical providers willing to be paid for services at the network rates. As for Medicaid, expanding eligibility did not expand the participating physicians.

Narrow Care Networks

Plans offered through a state Health Insurance Exchange do not cover out-of-network care, except in emergency, which often means no coverage. These "narrow" networks are claustrophobic.

Each insurance carrier uses propriety data, propriety algorithms, to decide which providers can be in its narrow network. This lacks transparency, and it disregards existing patient-physician relationships. Is cost the only criterion? What of quality or efficiency?

For example, Empire Blue Cross Blue Shield created the narrow "Pathways" network for its 2014 offering by excluding all academic medical centers in New York City, such as Sloan Kettering, plus all the physicians associated with those institutions. For 2015, Empire broadened its network, but that could shrink in the future. The only insurer offering products on New Hampshire's exchange, Anthem Blue Cross BlueShield excluded ten of the state's 26 hospitals. Hospitals are included or excluded based on care unit price.

These narrow networks usually are state-specific. You can't cross state lines for covered care, even if your insurance company sells the product in every state. You may not know this until care is needed, or after it's obtained, increasing your economic risk.

Who fits in these "chosen" networks is a source of confusion and mystery to patients and physicians alike. Health plans do not make it easy. Network and product names constantly change, and so do the rules for participating physicians.

UnitedHealthcare has products called Core, Metro and Charter. Physicians participating in networks called Freedom and Liberty do not participate in these products unless a patient is in a hospital, and *if* the physician is participating. How is a physician or a patient to keep this nuance clear? Confused patients get surprise bills.

Verifying if your physician is in a narrow network is a challenge by itself. Reviews of the online directories by the health plans have revealed high degrees of inaccuracy, like the availability of a listed physicians, who's really not accepting new patients. *The Los Angeles Times* in 2014 reported 12 percent of the physicians in Anthem's online directory for California were not accepting new patients, and 25 percent of the office locations were inaccurate.

'You Can Keep Your Current Plan'

"If you like your current health insurance plan, you can keep it." Well, this politic statement by President Obama needed an asterisk, too. You can keep your plan *if* it meets federal requirements.

The ACA set up essential benefits that all health insurance plans must cover. If your current health insurance plan did not include all these essential benefits, it was not approved under the ACA.

Non-conforming policies get labeled as "junk policies" because of large gaps in the health benefits. Junk policies do satisfy the needs and finances of younger, healthier purchasers, who care about affordability more than benefits. A single male doesn't need maternity benefits, for instance, so 66 percent of male purchasers chose that cost savings, according to Healthcare.org.

ACA Bronze, Silver, Gold, and Platinum plans. Not all that glitters is good.

However, coverage limits in junk policies often are not discovered until the excluded care is most needed, creating economic burdens for these patients, perhaps medical debt for them and their care providers.

In fairness to the ACA, it makes sense to set minimum standards on what must be covered under any health insurance policy.

The Trump administration let states accept non-conforming policies on their exchanges, those plans with less coverage and lower premiums. Excluding coverage for mental health, substance abuse treatment or maternity care does reduce premiums. Why pay a high premium for services you do not expect to use? Short-term savings on premiums may be regretted long-term when superior coverage is needed. One needs to balance costs and risks.

ACA Metallic Plans and Medical Debt

More than 60 percent of the personal bankruptcies in this nation relate to medical bills and the economic stress on families and individuals by the cost of care. The ACA was designed to address this tragedy, but does it really solve the problem?

Bronze, Silver, Gold, and Platinum insurance plans. Not all that glitters is good. Each metallic plan label carries a different level of patient financial responsibility. No ACA metallic plan by any name offers full protection from medical debt and financial ruin.

Here's a 2019 overview (thanks Kaiser Family Foundation).

• *Bronze Plans* — Affordable Premiums cover only 60 percent of approved medical costs, so 40 percent of costs is the responsibility of patients and their families. Annual deductibles average $3,154 for individuals and $6,258 for families.

• *Silver Plans* — Less affordable premiums cover 70 percent. Deductibles average $2,188 for individuals, and $4,375 for families.

• *Gold Plans* — More pricey premiums cover 80 percent. Deductibles average $667 for individuals, and $1,335 for families.

• *Platinum Plans* — High premiums cover 90 percent. Annual deductibles average $25 for individuals and $50 for families.

Limits on out-of-pocket (OOP) costs vary by state Marketplace, based on premium levels. A marketing twist gives plan consumers a choice of their own deductible and OOP limits, based on premiums. Offerings on ACA exchanges vary state-to-state.

On average, as of 2019, the least costly Bronze plans capped out-of-pocket at $6,350 for individuals and $12,700 for families. Silver plans capped OOP at $5,500 for individuals, $11,000 for families. People with modest incomes trying to save on monthly premiums stand a high risk personal or family economic devastation.

Covid invited insurance to reassess their ACA plan deductibles and OOP caps, but I can report no big shifts by late 2021. As always, the higher the premium, the greater the coverage, the less personal financial responsibility. So, pay higher monthly premiums, or pay when services are needed? It's a choice, but not a great one.

Patient financial responsibility is not eliminated under the ACA. The public is lulled into a false sense of security. Deductibles can be hefty. They come just as illness or injury is reducing family income. As patient's financial responsibility goes up, so does the provider's risk of non-payment, and its likelihood. Medical debt remains a real problem for all, patients and care providers alike.

Care coverage is not guaranteed, even if a provider verifies coverage at the time of care. individuals who purchase coverage on an exchange are granted a grace period to pay their monthly insurance premium. Until a premium is 90 days overdue, care providers may be told a patient is covered, only to have that claim denied.

About a fifth of those buying policies on ACA exchanges default before the end of their grace period. This leaves the provider stuck with collecting their medical debt, or absorbing it.

The ACA removed barriers to buying health insurance, removed prohibitions on preexisting conditions, provided plan coverage for children up to age 26 on a family plan, made healthcare insurance available to individuals without employer-provided plans, and expanded Medicaid availability. All this, plus premium subsidies, increased affordability for a large segment of the middle class.

Patient financial responsibility is not eliminated under the ACA.

The ACA overall has resulted in a decrease of the total number of uninsured people. Kaiser Family Foundation found the number of non-elderly uninsured Americans fell from 44 million in 2013 (the year before ACA) to fewer than 28 million uninsured in 2016. However, after the Trump Administration's 2017 elimination of the sanctions enforcing the individual mandate, plus fresh restrictions on Medicaid eligibility, the uninsured rate rose from 7.5 percent to 8.5 percent by 2018, according to the US Census Bureau.

Kaiser and other healthcare watchers warn the affordability of insurance policies remains a core issue. High costs are the principal reason most often cited by those who remain uninsured.

Patient Responsibility and Transparency

One gospel for constraining the inflationary spiral of health care costs is the idea of "patient engagement." This consumerism term actually means more money out of the patient's pocket. People with economic "skin-in-the-game" are expected to change their behavior from passive patients into fully engaged consumers. Patients are expected to consider their own needs and press their providers for more economical care, wisely choosing their care providers on the basis of quality and affordability.

Insured patients absorbing the higher cost of care, as consumers, seek to know their cost for all services. They care little about what their plan will pay care providers. They care what it will cost them out-of-pocket for their encounters with the health system.

In theory, this is consumerism at its best, so costs are a factor in choosing the care provided and the actual provider of that care, plus the location for care services. In a life-threatening situation, care is always sought. Price is a secondary thought. In an elective situation, the smart consumer will be just that, smart and thrifty.

Insured patients are responsible for all costs until they satisfy their deductible, but deductibles only begin the costs passed along to patients. Kaiser Family Foundation analyzed the Truven Health Analytics *MarketScan* database of commercial claims and care encounters for ACA Bronze, Silver and Gold plans from 2006 to 2016. They found deductibles were about 51 percent of the costs that patients bore. Other forms of cost sharing left patient paying upwards of 30 percent or more of the total cost of their care under ACA plans. Cost sharing is even greater in 2021.

The worthy ideal of informed consumers misses a key ingredient — *transparency*. Personal responsibility is hampered if patients cannot learn the cost of care before services are rendered.

Pricing transparency is not a regular consideration of the health care industry. But without transparency, patients cannot be engaged consumers — voting with their wallets in seeking the most cost-effective care providers. Without transparency, a patient is readily victimized by the complexity of health care providers billing and contracting practices.

Transparency is among the last things desired by the health care industry. Historically, it's not been necessary. Health plan payments rates were between the provider and insurer, after the deductible. What was charged to your health plan was the result of the best marketplace negotiations that the hospital or other provider could maximize. After the patient paid affordable deductibles, and some copayments, it did not matter to the patient what deal a hospital or physician cut for reimbursement. The entire process was obscured behind a screen.

> The ideal of informed consumers misses a key ingredient — *transparency*. Personal responsibility as consumers is hampered if patients cannot learn the true cost of care before services are rendered.

Hospitals and other care providers offer a public retail price list for services, called a "chargemaster." No one pays "retail" except for the uninsured self-pay patients, who seldom can afford the list price. Insurance companies pay the negotiated contract rates, discounted from the price list. Medicare and Medicaid pay formula-based reimbursements. Actual payments are different than the list prices. With this level of complexity, health care providers are ill-prepared for the "conscious consumer" patient seeking to shop prices.

More importantly, providers don't want their contracted rates revealed. They believe that if their negotiated rates are disclosed, insurers paying higher rates will seek to reduce their payments. They believe that if patients know the likely price, especially the cost before receiving elective services, patients would actually become more engaged consumers, voting with their wallets.

No provider wants to compete on price. True transparent pricing might force hospitals to prove they really do provide a superior product, to justify their charges or lose their patient volume. Most care providers think it's far better to keep on promoting their high quality without ever truly having to authenticate it.

Transparency was advanced by a Trump Administration executive order, "Improving Price and Quality Transparency in American Healthcare to Put Patients First." Centers for Medicare & Medicaid Services (CMS) finalized this order as a policy in November 2019. The intent was creating a patient-driven healthcare system by requiring hospitals to make the

> The new CMS 'Hospital Price Transparency' final rule went into effect on January 1, 2021, but still 94% of hospitals are non-compliant. They accept the low fines as a cost of doing business.

prices for items and services more transparent, so patients can be more informed about what they might pay for hospital services. One month later, the American Hospital Association responded with a federal lawsuit to block these policies.

Trying to stake out the high ground, AHA claimed transparency will not drive down prices, but it will raise them. Open pricing will drive providers in a community to increase their rates to match the highest-charging provider, not the lowest one. Think of gas stations at the same corner matching prices.

The hospitals' suit took a position common in opposing public transparency. Over-abundance of information will be too confusing for patients to understand. It's the same excuse hospitals have long made against releasing data, like caesarian section rates or surgical infection rates. "Trust us because we care about you."

Nothing prohibits a forward-looking hospital from voluntarily calculating their insurance reimbursements and giving patients a guaranteed pre-service price. In actual fact, I can name no hospital wanting to expose themselves to the risk of being wrong about the price, or worse, risk the paying patient going elsewhere.

The new CMS "Hospital Price Transparency" final rule went into effect on January 1, 2021. The opposing lawsuit by AHA and other national organizations failed, and court appeals are pending.

As for hospital industry compliance, PatientsRightsAdvocate.org reported 94 percent of hospitals were still non-compliant by June 2021. Hospitals remain non-compliant and not transparent. They accept the rather low federal fines as a cost of doing business.

For you as a responsible patient, if care is not an emergency, ask or demand up-front pricing. Join the growing chorus. For inpatient care, your local hospital may have a monopoly on beds. For out-patient care, seek and compare prices from the local non-hospital providers. The savings can be exceptional. Self advocate.

The ACA is Really Insurance Reform

A key provision of the ACA turned health insurance companies into public utilities, and thus regulated their profitability. Insurance products must pay out 85 percent (80 percent for the small group policies) for medical services, leaving 15 to 20 percent for administration and profits. If any more is spent on clams, insurance companies must adsorb the loss. if the medical expenses are lower than the 85 to 80 percent levels. any savings must be refunded to the insured. Profitability is not what it was for insurance companies.

The cost of health insurance is still tied to the cost of care — unit cost per service provided, and the volume of services. There's been little change. From 2008 to 2016, health plan costs increased by 50 percent, reflected in higher insurance premiums paid by employers and the higher payroll deductions of employees.

> The ACA did not change the fundamental structure for financing care. It did not end medical debt.

Employers offset the increases by applying the deductible models of the ACA marketplace plans. If anything, the ACA legitimized and reintroduced the deductible as a major tool for shifting the cost of medical care to the patient. By 2016, *Money* magazine reports, deductibles above $1,000 were standard, and 51 percent of insured employees were exposed to high out-of-pocket costs.

The ACA did not change the fundamental structure for delivery of medical care. It did not change the care financing model of fee-for-service. It did not move hospitals to communities where they're most needed. It did not produce more primary care physicians, nor enhance ambulatory options. It did not end medical debt.

Re-engineering care delivery has been left up to the healthcare industry, which has proven itself to be dedicated to protecting the status quo and their bottom line rather than adopting reforms that meet evolving local community medical needs.

I believe that insurance is the wrong way to finance healthcare. We cannot end medical debt without addressing the oo structures driving high health care costs. We need to rethink our approach.

Financing Healthcare in a Pandemic

Health insurance policies often have an interesting limitation — exclusions for injury or illness resulting from an act of war, declared or undeclared, like in a terrorist attack. Such circumstances would likely push health insurers beyond their financial reserves. But what happens during a public health crisis? The Covid pandemic was not anticipated by most health insurance companies, but for them, the pandemic has been among the best of times.

To see why this is so, consider how health insurance companies like the month of February. They receive 30 days of premiums with exposure to claims for 28 days (or 29 days in leap years). Curiously, federal pay for Covid dramatically reduced the insurance companies' exposure. The hospitals curtailed elective services, and the patients voluntarily curtailed accessing health care providers. For health insurers, this has meant earning the same premiums with greatly reduced exposure for costs.

> I believe that insurance is the wrong way to finance healthcare.

At one point in my career, I offered physicians and hospitals the opportunity to be compensated on a "capitation" basis, that is, paid a percent of insurance premiums regardless of volume. This model was widely rejected by medical providers, who preferred to retain pay-as-you-do fees for services provided. I can only imagine that as the pandemic hit, when patient volume fell for all other medical services, some hospital CEOs and physicians might be thinking that capitation may not be such a bad idea. A piece of all premiums, not tied to services provided, could help the specialists not needed for Covid care, like surgeons.

Covid confirmed the fallacy of fee-for-service as a means of financing the healthcare system.

Covid confirmed the fallacy of fee-for-service as a means of financing the health care system and its providers. Coping with Covid demands has meant that revenue disappeared or shifted from the usual mix of patients and pay-sources, yet the providers were expected to be there "at the ready," as usual. If a community fire department, on standby 24/7, was paid only when they battle a burning building, would the community assure sufficient financing for the fire department by waiving all the building codes and fire safety regulations as strategy to bolster the demand for paid firefighting? That's absurd.

The same can be said of financing a healthcare system based on illness and injury. Efforts to reduce the need for care are not prominent in health planning. If the goal is health, is financing healthcare only by fees-for-services the best we can do as a society?

PART II

Forgiving
Medical Debt

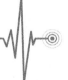

Money is better than poverty,
if only for financial reasons.

— WOODY ALLEN

CHAPTER 8

Debt is in the Details

Craig Antico

When I co-created RIP Medical Debt in 2014 with my partner and co-author, Jerry Ashton, our purpose was and has always been to achieve a forthright, big audacious goal: Raise money to buy unpaid and unpayable medical debt, and then forgive that debt to benefit the neediest debtors. On the surface, simple enough.

In performing this service, we've learned the truth of the saying, "The devil is in the details." It exactly fits our work and our mission. That simple. That hard. People tell us they love the goal of removing medical debt burdens from distressed people who need and deserve charitable debt relief. Our donors, partners and sponsors naturally want and need to understand the details, as may you.

Precisely what does RIP Medical Debt do? How do we go about locating, qualifying and cancelling medical debt? Where and how is medical debt located? Who owns someone's personal medical debt, and how does that come about? When does medical debt enter the "secondary debt" market? Why is so much medical debt still owed? Does medical debt ever go away? Is it really a hardship? Why?

To answer these questions, I need to tell you a bit more about RIP. We saw early the need for a "business case" that resonated with donors: Forgive as much unpayable medical debt as we can.

As two former collections industry executives, we were uniquely positioned to raise public awareness about how medical debt harms millions of Americans and our nation. We found people agreed that unpayable medical debt is a wrong that needs correcting. They'd be upset that healthcare costs are the leading cause of bankruptcies, causing 15 million people and their families to go insolvent annually. The more people learned, the more they wanted to help.

This public response is why RIP has exceeded our initial goal of abolishing $1 billion in medical debt. As of this new edition, RIP has forgiven $5 billion for millions of individuals. Is this big news? It's a drop in the ocean. Can we do more? If so, how?

Well, let's get into those devilish details.

Does Medical Debt Ever End?

If you owe a relative or friend money that you promised to pay back, do you imagine that debt ever goes away? Fifteen years from now, any unpaid debt lingers between you, so you may isolate yourself from that person. You may feel anxious, guilty, ashamed, upset, or disappointed that you could not, would not, did not know how, or are plain unwilling to pay them back. From a legal standpoint, the debt is still owed. Even after the :statute of limitations" expires, ethically, the debt remains due. A promise is a promise.

Exchange your friend for a hospital or any medical care provider. Does a bill you owe ever go away? No. You have only four options:

1. You or another can pay the medical debt in-full or settle it.
2. The provider can issue a credit to eliminate the debt.
3. The debt can be "discharged" by a U.S. bankruptcy court.
4. The debt can be "extinguished" by law as a voided contract.

Those are your four options. Unless one of those events occurs, you still owe a debt until the day you die, but then only if your estate is insolvent, or if you don't live in one of nine U.S. states where debt is inherited. Generally, medical debt never goes away.

What if a hospital told you they wrote off your bill as bad debt? What if they changed their billing system and stopped sending you statements? What if a doctor will accept the amount your insurance pays? What if that bill is 15 or 20 years old? Sorry. Most likely, your medical bill is still owed.

Is this ethical or morally right? Realistically, can any debt be valid if those owing it, no matter how hard they work to be personally responsible, can never pay it back in their lifetime? This is the sorry reality with medical debt.

Whom can we all blame for the egregious injustice and burden of medical debt? Shall we blame the "healthcare system," the creditors, care providers, or loan originators, the government? Do we blame the patients, blame the victims? Laying blame is no solution.

> Can any debt be valid if those owing it, no matter how hard they work to be personally responsible, can never pay it back in their lifetime?

To eliminate that onus, in my view, some unpayable debt in the health care system should be extinguished, canceled, as if it never existed in the first place. I hope for a day when medical debt does not thrust people into hardship or worse. Until then, debt is debt. RIP will keep contacting medical debt owners to find all the debt we can buy and abolish. It's our "fairness doctrine."

Debt companies contact RIP offering to sell us their "receivables" or "assets" — what your debts are to them. Knowing debt never dies and government constantly shifts the playing field, some call us to protect their patients, their customers (or themselves) from liability for future collections. They know that if their debt company goes bankrupt, a trustee can use their superpowers to demand payment from all debtors, no matter how old are the debts.

'Zombie' debt is a debt that bounces from agency to agency, from debt buyer to debt buyer, and never dies.

In our industry, "zombie" debt is a debt that bounces from agency to agency, from debt buyer to debt buyer, and never dies. Too often, a third-party debt collector convinces a hospital or provider to place all of their oldest unpaid accounts with them, promising they will only charge a collection fee for those bills if they collect. That old debt now gets new life. Patients who thought their bills were dead suddenly start getting collection calls.

What if you default on that creditor and stop calling? Once they exhaust all their collection activity and mark you as a loss, they may formally forgive the debt or settle it in part. Whew! You think the debt is no longer owed, but there's a catch.

The government considers the amount you did not have to pay as ordinary income. The creditor sends you a 1099-C, "Cancellation of Debt Income," with a copy to the IRS. You must pay taxes on that "income." For instance, the U.S. government annually forgives $110 billion in student loan debt. The "lucky" ones get a 1099-C.

You could owe taxes for income you never saw.

Unintended Consequences

Medical debt never goes away, not legally or ethically, not as a burden on people's minds. Medical debt is a hardship. That is why RIP seeks to buy and cancel as much medical debt as possible (what we call "debt of necessity"), no matter its age or legal status.

To show what we deal with at RIP, take the statute of limitations. States have an "out-of-statute" time limit on when a creditor can collect money owed through a lawsuit (or the threat of one). This can range from two or three years to more than 10 years. You may think that after the statutory time limit is over, collections stop, and the debt is extinguished. That is a common misperception.

Some states go further to protect consumers. Mississippi altered its statue of limitations so debts are automatically extinguished after three years. If this law becomes common, I'd expect to see a sharp turn in the way hospitals charge their customers, and how quickly they collect medical bills. If consumer protection laws or regulations limit the time in which creditors can collect on a bill, the inevitable "unintended consequences" might be disastrous.

If we end people's ability to pay credit (medical debt) over time, and demand payment upfront in cash, expect access to healthcare (or any service or product) to be severely impacted.

One result could be a wide "outsourcing" of care financing away from care providers, which disconnects patient-doctor relationships. Outsourced medical bills then would be owed to a finance company or bank, not the provider, as if you used a credit card. If you must pay medical bills up front, in fact, won't you use credit cards? High interest credit cards are *not* the way to pay medical bills.

Imagine what would happen if hospitals were "forced" to bring credit finance companies into their hospitals. It's possible patients would owe banks at least $800 billion a year.

Only 10 percent of medical debt is reported to credit bureaus, tallying $75 billion. This would change. Banks, by law and industry standards, would be required to report all that $800 billion to credit bureaus. This would appear on reports as "other" consumer credit, not as medical debt. Credit cards buy big-screen TVs and vacations, right? Not so! We estimate at least a third of the almost $900 billion owed on credit cards is for medical OOP expenses.

People with medical debt on their credit reports already have about 70 percent more credit card debt than those without medical debt. Mississippi's experiment could cause finance company or bank takeovers of medical billing. Beware of unintended consequences from the most well-intentioned healthcare regulations.

Uncollectable Medical Bills

When hospitals cannot collect on accounts owed by individuals who are qualified for charity care or Medicaid (but did not sign up), that's vexing to both the hospital and the collection agent.

Hospitals collect unpaid bills internally if they have the means to do so, but accounts are often placed for collection to comply with regulations. These accounts likely will become "bad debt."

To retain a 501(c)(3) status, hospitals needs to meet Community Benefit Requirements. A hospital must show the U.S. government they're supporting the needy and those in hardship. However, at least 30 percent of the accounts assigned for collections should have qualified for charity car, in my experience, one shared by others in the medical debt industry. A hospital's "account misclassification" problem becomes another unintended consequence of regulations intended to protect healthcare consumers.

Hospitals cannot sell to debt buyers the accounts that collection agencies declare as uncollectible. Hospitals must take the "hit." That hardly resolves the debt problem for patients. They enter purgatory.

Although the hospital appears to have stopped collecting on the old debt, the patients still know they owe for care.

These debts makes up the lion's share of all medical bills owed by consumers that have gone to third-party collections. This is where we come in at RIP as debt buyers and forgivers.

How is Medical Debt Bought and Sold?

To understand how RIP is able to abolish debt, you need to see how it's bought by debt buyers, investors, to make money.

Medical billing accounts you owe, like mortgages, can be bought and sold. At a profit, of course. Collection executives recover money for a living. Debt-buying executives who invest in a debt portfolio need to buy debt at a price where they can profit, collecting two to three times the amount they pay. If they buy a portfolio of debt for $10,000, for instance, they expect to collect $20,000 to $30,000.

> Medical billing accounts, like mortgages, can be bought and sold. At a profit, of course.

All hospitals and most physicians use collection agencies to help collect money owed by their patients after the insurance company paid its portion. Hospitals staff the big collection departments so that each collector has 8,000 accounts to handle at any given point in time. Staff overwhelm leads to long-unpaid accounts being placed with third-party collection agencies. The Association of Credit and Collection Professionals International says there are 100,000 bill collectors in the USA, and more than half of them collect medical debt.

Suppose a local hospital uses the same collection agency as a debt buyer. The hospital asks, why wait for the agency to collect when the debt buyer offer cash? A business needs cash to operate. After all, "accounts receivable" are not cash unless collected.

Debt buyers bring needed capital to health care providers, who need not wait two, three or four years to finally get their money, if ever. Debt buyers are sophisticated with strong dispute resolution skills and sophisticated collection practices. There's just no room in their world any more for previous unethical practices, not like we've heard about. The debt industry, as a whole, has shifted to treating debtors with respect.

> # The debt industry, as a whole, has shifted to treating debtors with respect

Debt bought from hospitals is seldom bought for the low prices RIP pays. Prices are closer to five, ten or 15 cents on the dollar. Price depends on the age of the billing accounts, the likelihood of contacting patients successfully, and the likelihood of collecting from them. As a business, debt buyers take on such risk, aware they might *not* collect two to three times the amount they paid.

If a debt buyer pays $50 for each $1,000 bill owed, for example, they must collect $150 to $200 per $1,000, on average, to make an acceptable return for the risk assumed by them, their bankers and investors. They may collect on "fresh" accounts quickly, yet it can take three to ten years to collect from the remaining accounts — three to ten years of phone calls, letters, and even lawsuits.

More than seven percent of all workers in the USA have income garnishments. Most are for child support or alimony, yet more than 25 percent of those garnishments are from medical debt judgments. Medical debt supports the entire debt industry.

Hospital Community Benefit Requirements

Charity care is only one required community benefit a hospital offers its patients in return for state and federal tax exemptions. Hospitals can lose their federal tax exemptions if they do not comply with community benefit requirements. charitable hospitals obtain significant benefits by complying with IRS and state regulations.

On average, hospitals spend about six percent of their revenues on improving the health of their community. At the 2020 start of the Covid pandemic, providers contributed much greater than six percent of their revenues, to their credit and fiscal loss.

Part tax-exempt hospitals proving that they provide community benefits is documentation of initiatives, activities, and investments they've undertaken to improve health within the community.

Community benefit requirements offer opportunities. Distilled from research by Plante Moran, here 's an overview:

• *Community Assessment* — The hospital must conduct a local "Community Health Needs Assessment" (CHNA), and adopt an "implementation plan" addressing the needs. This must be submitted every three years. The strategic plan must be adopted on or before the 15th day of the fifth month after the year a CHNA is conducted. A $50,000 excise fine curbs non-compliance.

• *Charity Care Policy* — The hospital must create a Financial Assistance Policy (FAP), publicized within the community.

• *Emergency Care Policy* — The hospital must create an emergency Policy for providing care without regard to FAP eligibility.

• *Billing Limits* — The hospital must limit amounts charged under the FAP to no more than that billed to insured patients.

• *Collection Limits* — The hospital is prohibited from collection actions against patients without first checking FAP eligibility.

Tax-exempt hospitals report four items on their Schedule H to document how they are benefiting their communities:

1. Financial assistance and means-tested government programs.
2. Community building activities.
3. Medicare shortfall fiscal report.
4. Bad debt attributable to charity care.

Meeting the community benefit requirements in 2011 alone was worth $24.6 billion, noted Project HOPE. That tax exemption (state and federal) was shared by 60 percent of 5,500 U.S. hospitals.

What if hospitals could apply their bad debt from eligible charity care toward meeting their Community Benefit Requirements?

What if hospitals could apply their bad debt for eligible charity care toward meeting their Community Benefit Requirements? Based on hospital IRS tax returns in 2013, this exceeded $67 billion, reported the Healthcare Financial Management Association, which in 2018 placed hospital bad debt at $56.5 billion. American Hospital Association reported $702 billion in "uncompensated care" in 2000 for 40 percent of all U.S. hospitals. It's higher now.

What if the billions in bad debt are written off as tax exemptions? Is hospital leadership ready to do this? A culture of care and charity starts at the top. Senior executives and governing boards can make change happen. Is the business of healthcare distracting them from their mission of health?

RIP provides an effective and sane way for hospitals to rid their books of medical debt, a "safe harbor" to end intractable problems from medical debt. Based on recent Schedule 990 H forms publicly filed by tax-exempt hospitals, the potential is at least $25 billion!

Everyone knows hospital bad debt is owed. Letting debt "sit on the books" doesn't make it go away, nor does it grant healthy peace of mind to those owing medical debt they cannot pay.

Community hospitals are not equipped with the cost accounting systems, analytics and reporting to provide reliable evidence that they do provide care for the needy. We are certain hospitals provide this community benefit, but they have a hard time coming up with systems-generated evidence to prove it.

Working in partnership with RIP's analytics, leveraging our tax-exempt charity status, hospitals can provide their communities with the miracle of medical debt forgiveness with no tax consequences for patients. The only "debt details" left to manage will be identifying the accounts to cancel and asking RIP to do the rest.

The cure for medical debt is in the details, for goodness' sake.

Which Debt Does RIP Buy?

We at RIP can cost-effectively buy portfolios of accounts from medical providers and debt buyers because we research accounts deeper than they do. We are debt buyers who are not economically constrained by profit. We care only about the social profit.

Our strategic partner, TransUnion Healthcare, believes in what we're doing. We use their data, publicly available data and purchased data to evaluate portfolios, valuing our likely impact for qualifying individuals in a portfolio, making an offer to buy it, and then closing the deal. We buy the debt causing the most hardship.

Within the bounds of HIPPA, we get the best possible picture of patients in the context of their debts and situations. With this data, we can better price a portfolio and assess the benefit of debt cancellation. We do this not to ensure our donors don't overpay, but to ensure that the people who most need help get our debt relief. We become, essentially, debtors' second-chance safety net.

Sometimes we locate debt and go find a donor. Sometimes we find a donor and then locate debt. We may seek a medical provider willing to sell us their bad debt. It's variable. For instance, a donor in Southwestern Virginia made a significant pledge to wipe out hardship debt in his region. With money from this donor and other donors, in 2021 RIP bought from Ballad Health $278 million worth of bad debt, assisting 82,000 people in Tennessee and Virginia.

> Our work is the reverse of a collection agency. RIP cancels the debt in full, no strings. We then make sure the credit blemish is removed.

We'll also buy medical debt on the secondary debt market. We run located debt through our analytics, so we are confident about buying only accounts that qualify for our charity work. We then negotiate a price for a portfolio and take possession by paying for it.

As the legal owners of a debt, we can legitimately cancel it. extinguish it. As a 501(c)(3) charity, RIP's debt forgiveness does not count as taxable income to the recipient.

What we do with debt differs from what collection agencies do. Penniless accounts, for collectors, are nuisances they park on credit reports on the chance one day the debtor gets a job or inheritance or wins the lottery, so monies appear to pay off the bill, just to clear the debt from credit reports, be done with it once and for all.

RIP buys older medical billing account portfolios from hospitals and debt sellers at a steep discount from the amount originally owed to the medical providers, usually for pennies on the dollar.

From the date of portfolio purchase, our work is the reverse of a collection agency. RIP cancels the debt in full, no strings attached. We then make sure that the credit blemish is removed from credit reports. Within 90 days of RIP buying that bill, the medical debt vanishes as if it had never been owed.

Such debt purchases can only be done in volume. If RIP tried to purchase one account at a time, we'd have to pay 50 times the $5 to $15 we pay now for $1,000 in debt. This is why our charity cannot forgive debt for any single individual. It's unfeasible now.

Our success comes only from partnerships with donors and debt sellers. Medical debt relief occurs when we join with those who want to free their fellow humans from undue destructive circumstances. No judgment, no pity. Just a gift, one stranger to another.

Also important is a hospital, doctor or debt owner willing to sell or donate accounts to us, rather than continuing to collect internally or parking bills on credit reports. Imagine the pleasure of a hospital or provider after donating, or selling for pennies, something of little value in return for genuinely improving people's lives.

We and our "social investor" donors agree. A collection process that takes three to ten years to complete is too long and too socially damaging. We aim to remove hardship from debtors by taking the bill collector and debt buyer out of the picture by the second or third year of an unpaid bill. We work through the market pricing system, not through legislation. Our business experience and relationships enable us to take hardship medical debt off the street.

First-Hand Material Hardship

Medical debt has had a big impact on my own family's finances. During the first five years of RIP Medical Debt's existence, my family experienced a period of prolonged poverty with major out-of-pocket expenses due to illness and material hardship.

Two years after Jerry and I started RIP in 2014, my spouse asked me a hard question: "Why are we going into debt to get other people out of debt?" I had look clearly at what I was doing.

The answers I gave my wife were not an explanation based on logic or self-preservation. I had to seek advice from friends to help resolve this in myself. My determination to keep going was against my family obligations as a provider. My pastor helped with my dilemma. I'm grateful my family persevered in tough times.

Two years after starting RIP in 2014, my spouse asked me, "Why are we going into debt to get other people out of debt?"

To withstand my not having income for almost three years despite all of my hard work, we lived on my wife's income as a teaching assistant. We used up all our savings. We sold our home and used the proceeds. We rented for half of what we'd paid for the mortgage. Some education for our children had to be delayed. My credit report rating fell.

Thank God we had health insurance. From all the chronic stress of financial uncertainty, my wife entered the hospital. To pay bills, we hocked all of her family jewelry and silver. (I am grateful to say I returned my wife's precious family heirloom, thanks to RIP's earning enough after John Oliver to pay me a basic salary.)

During that period, my family incurred "debt of necessity" three times our household income. Try to imagine the hardship of living for years in poverty with a family of six, no savings, and you are in your mid-fifties? Our income fell to below two times the federal poverty level. Plainly put, we were insolvent. We had out-of-pocket medical expenses and debt equal to more than five percent of the family gross annual income. By RIP's criteria, the Antico family was qualified for RIP's debt forgiveness!

This is not a victim story. It's my narrative of what it took for RIP to exist and start to flourish. Compared to the tales of hardship we read in letters and emails arriving at RIP daily, the Antico family had it easy. (Don't tell my wife I wrote that.)

Was putting my family in jeopardy for RIP the right thing to do? Rationally, no. But forgiving debt is what I *had* to do. Jerry made his own sacrifices while RIP lived on his credit cards. We both went into personal debt. Why? We could not in good conscience walk away from the massive mountain of medical debt that our backgrounds made us uniquely equipped to help conquer.

Where else in the world could you ever hope to find two former collections industry executives willing to reverse their career course, deciding not to collect medical debt but to forgive it?

More than two years in, by the time of the John Oliver show in June 2016, RIP had reached a level of forgiving almost $40 million in medical debt for 30,000 individuals who otherwise could never pay off those bills. We could not and would not stop.

Our personal finances stank, and we never got rich, but we were hooked on abolishing medical debt.

*There is scarcely anything
that drags a person down like debt.*

— P. T. Barnum

CHAPTER 9

The John Oliver Effect:
Gifts and Lessons

Jerry Ashton

Perhaps the first time you heard anything about medical debt was in 2016 when HBO's "Last Week Tonight with John Oliver" did a segment on debt buyers. To expose how ridiculously easy it is to buy and collect old debt, the show spent $60,000 to buy a batch of uncollectable medical billing accounts, a portfolio with a face value close to $15 million.

Rather than collect on that debt, John Oliver in the live studio pushed a big button to signal donating all of it to RIP Medical Debt, briefly displaying the logo of our startup charity. We then canceled the unpaid healthcare bills of nearly 9,000 people in Texas — the largest single giveaway in American television history. His viewers were enthralled. RIP was transformed.

Overnight, RIP became a "hot" news story. Overnight, donations began flowing in (plus moving debt relief pleas). Please appreciate that in the two years since 2014 when Craig Antico, Robert Goff and I co-founded RIP, we'd barely brought in $50,000 in donations.

Because RIP can buy older debt portfolios from debt sellers for about a penny on the dollar, by then we'd been able to purchase and forgive about $5 million in debt. That amount was eclipsed in one day. The surge of donations let us abolish tens of millions in unpaid medical bills causing personal and family hardship.

RIP began receiving requests and proposals for debt forgiveness campaigns by community groups, labor unions, churches, veterans, high school students, philanthropists, and others. We discovered amazing local, regional and national allies who care about ending medical debt. We've grown the staff and added consultants. We've expanded and refined our operations.

As a result of such activity and accompanying local to national media attention, by time the first edition of this book was published in January 2018, donations to RIP had relieved almost $1 billion in medical debt for struggling individuals and families.

As we go to press with this new edition in autumn 2021, RIP has just passed a milestone of $5 billion in debt relief. A major landmark and national first is that we've recently begun acquiring bad debt directly from hospitals, which opens more possibilities.

As part of our mission, RIP increasingly participates in public policy discussions about the healthcare system's structure and financing. Within our bounds as a nonprofit, we're helping to shift societal forces producing medical bills that people cannot pay. Most remarkable of all, our work benefits tens of millions of people.

Enter John Oliver

All of our charity growth flowed, literally, from a few moments of exposure on a popular satiric commentary show on HBO, hosted in New York City by a sharp British-born comedian. Our 15 seconds of fame caused an astounding change in fortune for our struggling little nonprofit. We call this "The John Oliver Effect."

As his fans know, John Oliver uses his national reach to expose the flaws and absurdities of politicians, extremists, miscreants, and industries unhinged from ethics or common sense. He also loves to elicit attention through outrageous acts of public service, which is how RIP entered the picture.

For a segment on debt buyers, John Oliver and his producers formed a debt-buying company that for about $60,000 bought a batch of bad debt with a face value near $15 million. For ethical and comedic purposes, they chose to forgive the debt in a splashy way. Oprah Winfrey set the standard on live TV in 2004. She gave away $8 million in new automobiles to the 276 members of her audience. "You get a car! You get a car! And you get a car!" Now John Oliver had $15 million to give away, so he would "out-Oprah Oprah."

> Our 15 seconds of fame caused an astounding change in fortune for our struggling little charity. We call this "The John Oliver Effect."

The HBO producer's challenge was forgiving the debt in a way that did not count as taxable income for the debtors, as with student loan forgiveness. For advice, they consulted a respected New York tax attorney. She told them they needed a tax-exempt charity with the expertise to responsibly meet the HIPAA "permissible use" rules for medical accounts.

As it happened on her desk sat a copy of a new book, *The Patient, The Doctor and The Bill Collector,* which I'd written with Robert Goff. As her client, Robert a few days earlier had gifted her a copy. She told the producers, "These are the people you need to see."

HBO called Robert, who referred them to Craig and me. We met at HBO's Manhattan offices. All the right people sat around a table. All the right questions were asked and answered. After the flurry of due diligence, a deal was done.

Last Week Tonight would donate to RIP Medical Debt the $15 million debt portfolio plus sufficient funds to process the accounts and mail out the forgiveness notification letters.

The show aired two weeks later on June 6, 2016.

Oliver started the famous "Debt Buyers" segment by lambasting the collections and debt buying industry. He revealed how readily personal hospital medical debt can be purchased and collected by almost anyone. He said it does not matter how old is the debt, nor how bad the financial condition of the debtor.

At the show climax, after Oliver had described his debt purchase, the RIP logo appeared above his right shoulder as he announced that he was donating the debt to "a 501(c)(3) charity, RIP Medical Debt, which will forgive this debt at no tax consequence to the recipient." He then walked to a stage and pushed a giant red button. Lights flashed. dollar bills fluttered down like confetti. Oliver lifted his arms, rejoicing "I am the new queen of daytime talk!"

Hundreds of people in his audience cheered. Thousands of posts hit the internet. Our website temporarily crashed from the crush of people wanting to learn more about this oddball charity that could — what was that again — forgive medical bills?

"The John Oliver Effect" and its lessons for us had begun.

Gifts and Lessons from Media Notice

We learned about our role in forwarding other's good actions, being the vehicle for people to make this world a better place. Our reward was sharing in all the publicity engendered by John Oliver's generosity. Good publicity attracts more publicity.

The John Oliver show stimulated donations quickly passing tens of thousands of dollars with commitments for far more. The most unexpected gifts were a flood of inquiries from individuals, organizations, special interest groups, and academia, all of whom desired to partner with RIP in some way. These gifts generated more public attention and taught us key lessons. Here are you five examples:

Gift 1 — Academic Interest (Get Smart People Interested)

Francis Wong, a doctoral student in the economics department at the University of California at Berkeley, was our first gift. Several days after the Oliver program aired, we received an email from him. He proposed an economic impact study on abolishing medical debt. His offer was immediately and enthusiastically accepted.

A week later, Ray Kluender, an economics doctoral student at MIT, made a similar request. We happily introduced Francis to Ray. (Have I mentioned we are great believers in collaboration?)

A month later, through Ray's influence, Craig and I were invited to the North America conference of J-PAL, the Abdul Latif Jameel

> They proposed an economic impact study on abolishing medical debt.

Poverty Action Lab at MIT. The global research center reduces poverty "by ensuring that policy is informed by scientific evidence." We were asked to present an explanation of RIP's work and mission as related to poverty alleviation. They also wanted to hear from two former bill collectors who were now forgiving debt.

After our short session, we were approached separately by Wes Yin, PhD, an associate professor of public policy at UCLA in Los Angeles, and by Neale Mahoney, PhD, assistant professor of economics at the University of Chicago. Like the grad students from UC/Berkeley and MIT, they wanted to do a medical debt economic impact study. Francis and Ray, meet Wes and Neale!

The four agreed to team up to conduct a study to be titled, "The Burden of Medical Debt and the Impact of Debt Forgiveness." Craig and I were in awe. Four outstanding academicians at four major universities formed a collaborative partnership with RIP to do first-ever research on the impact of medical debt forgiveness.

Fast forward: Three years into the study, in autumn 2020, as the team approached publication, they discussed their work at RIP's fifth annual Medical Debt Summit in New York, held virtually due to Covid. Their peer-reviewed paper later was published by *JAMA* in 2021. They proved unpayable medical debt has adverse impacts on individuals, families and society. We shift from theory to fact. (And congrats to Francis and Ray for earning your PhDs!)

Attending that online summit, were a rainbow array of leaders representing hospitals, physicians, patient advocates, collections, data technology, academia, government, NGOs, and philanthropy. We spotlighted the practical costs of unpayable healthcare debt and explored creative solutions. Held a month before the 2020 election, the summit did not make any newscast, but it affected those who participated. Who know what ripples may result?

Gift 2 — Technology Partners (Let a Techie Adopt You)

One/Zero Capital founder and CEO Vishal Garg and his team were intrigued by the John Oliver segment and reached out to us. Finding our work congruent with their corporate mission, which emphasizes social betterment, he invited RIP to share desk space at their offices in New York City. Office space was a big step up for us. We'd been working out of coffee shops and our homes, Craig in Rye and me in Manhattan. Robert joined us for board meetings.

One/Zero connected us to the TheNumber management team. They provided to us a data platform for locating and buying medical debt, plus a fast method to process accounts in large batches for debt forgiveness. Their technology, data scientists and team miraculously liberated Craig and I from manually processing the accounts that rising donations were letting RIP buy and forgive. Suddenly, we gained the infrastructure to cancel a lot more debt!

> Suddenly, we gained the infrastructure to cancel a lot more debt.

Fast Forward: RIP has benefited greatly from our relationship with the One/Zero family of companies. They capped off our fifth birthday in 2019 by giving us a check for $100,000 to fund our debt operations. I believe Vishal Garg's keen sense of social responsibility led him to support our work to benefit everyone in America.

We further partnered with TransUnion Healthcare. Their team helps us with data analytics of purchased debt portfolios to identify those in most need of help. They also play a pivotal role in removing cancelled accounts from the credit reports of the reporting agencies. We could not do what we do without them.

Gift #3 — The Doctor Is In (Find an Industry Ally)

We also attract in 2016 the partnership of a respected Southern California physician, Rishi Manchanda, MD. He wrote:

"Like many others, I imagine, I recently learned of your work through the John Oliver TV show. I am deeply interested in the intersection of health, financial security, literacy, and medical debt, especially for working families. I am active in advocacy and policy efforts to transform healthcare at local and national levels."

Dr. Manchanda, known for his TED talks, pioneered encouraging doctors to consider the "upstream" environmental and social conditions that contribute to sickness. He wanted to bring attention to the financial hardships that follow. We learned about the "social determinants" that generate medical debt in America.

> We learned about the 'social determinants' that generate medical debt.

"Resources that enhance quality of life can have a significant influence on population health outcomes," states the U.S. Office of Disease Prevention and Health Promotion. Among the resources are safe and affordable housing, access to education, public safety, availability of healthy foods, local emergency and medical services, and healthy community natural environments that are "free of life-threatening toxins."

He brought home to us how profoundly poverty means a lack of adequate shelter, good food and quality medical care. For those in poverty fortunate enough to afford healthy groceries, they may live in a "food desert" where fresh produce and unprocessed foods are simply not available, or they may live in a "transportation dessert," so they can't reach neighborhoods where better food is sold.

Dr. Manchanda at that time was chief medical officer of a large, privately owned and self-insured Southern California employer of migrant farm workers. In managing employee health clinics, he was seeking innovative ways to positively affect employee's upstream determinants to reduce the incidence of illness. In talking with his farmworker patients, he often heard about oppressive debt and bill collectors hounding them over unpaid medical bills.

To test the efficacy of debt forgiveness, his company donated $10,000 to fund a purchase of $2.1 million worth of medical debt in the rural area where his patients worked. While not intended as a proof of concept, this was the first time RIP rotated from "random act of kindness" to targeting a specific locale and population strata. This effort was a major breakthrough for RIP.

Dr. Manchanda subsequently left his employer to focus on his Studio City practice, Health Begins. Circling back to RIP in 2017, he led a community coalition of clinicians, advocates and academics that raised another $10,000 to abolish about $2 million in medical debt in Los Angeles and Ventura counties. Dr. Manchanda taught us that if we cannot remove people from locations with mountains of medical debt, we could begin to remove the mountain.

Fast forward: When Covid hit, Dr. Manchanda was among the healthcare leaders calling for a U.S. Community Health Care Corps, a modern version of the Depression era's Civil Conservation Corps. More community health means less medical debt.

Gift 4 — Student Philanthropists (Start Me Young)

Two Florida high school students, Samir Boussarhane and Falen McClellan, wrote to say they would emulate John Oliver and raise funds to abolish medical debt in their hometown, Pensacola. Could we help them? Of course!

Craig negotiated project terms with Pensacola High School for teacher oversight to ensure their efforts fit the requirements of the school's International Baccalaureate (IB) program.

The Pensacola Debt Sharks, as they called themselves, sought to raise the $10,000 needed to abolish $1 million in medical debt in the Pensacola and Mobile region. From pizza sales and after-school game nights, they earned local and national publicity. An anonymous donor stepped up with a generous contribution.

The pair and their allies finally raised more than $30,000, enough to abolish $3 million in unpaid medical bills. At a tribute the next year, Falen and Samir received the George Washington Community Award from the Freedoms Foundation at Valley Forge.

Fast Forward: Samir and Falen (now in college) paved the way for RIP's "Student Philanthropy" program with students around the country abolishing debt — despite Covid. New York high school students, for instance, erased $7 million in debt from their "Project Eraser" campaign. *Student-led programs are backed by RIP's Education and Engagement team.)

Their donation supported the largest single medical debt forgiveness campaign in U.S. history.

Charities of all sizes pray for a major donor, like a philanthropist, foundation or corporate sponsor. Major donors will make all of the difference between a charity barely getting by or becoming a robust force in their field. RIP he been blessed by such a gift.

A married couple with substantial means saw us on John Oliver and considered a donation. They checked us out through C-suite connections in Silicon Valley. Has anyone heard about this charity? Are these guys legit? Their search led them a San Francisco startup investor who told them RIP was doing a debt forgiveness campaign for his startup. He said we were all we said we were.

After more vetting and talking, RIP received a small contribution to open the relationship. What a relationship it's been! Choosing to be anonymous, in 2018 the pair made a seven-figure donation to RIP that let us buy and abolish $250 million in medical debt. The unprecedented donation rolled out in three stages.

The initial $150 million of relieved a block of $50 million in veterans and military debt. The next $50 million cancelled debt on Thanksgiving day. The last $50 million forgave debt during the December holidays. Their $250 million donation supported the largest single medical debt forgiveness campaign in U.S. history, helping 100,000 individuals and families in almost every state.

Fast Forward: RIP remains one of many important causes this couple supports. Some are much larger, and many are smaller. Each is carefully chosen and nurtured. RIP is in good company. We wish all charitable organization the same gift of good fortune.

Gift 5 — A Tidal Wave of Faith (Miracles Abound)

Ripples can become waves of awakening. In early 2018, Dallas broadcaster NBC-TV5 investigated local medical debt, which led to a campaign with RIP abolishing medical debt in thier broadcast area. They emulated stations around the country sponsoring community debt relief campaigns, primarily funded by their audiences. Local news stories featured debtors in the community who'd contacted RIP and agreed to tell their stories to the press. They went public (or stayed anonymous) to help others in their shoes.

We next received an email, from Covenant Church, a North Texas church with many campuses. They saw the Dallas news story and "wanted to work with RIP Medical Debt to pay off medical debt for families in North Texas."

Our back-and-forth calls and emails clarified for us at RIP the way to locate debt geographically and by need. Proposing initially a $50,000 contribution, Covenant instead donated $100,000 for debt relief. On Easter Sunday, 2018, pastor Stephen Hayes announced from the pulpit the "Good News" that the church was forgiving $10 million in medical debt. The event was covered by NBC-TV5 for a featured story on their nightly newscast.

Pastor Hayes told the reporter that the church invests $100,000 monthly in mailings to attract new members for their growing and diverse congregation. "Historically, a lot of churches have done it — where you spend upwards of six figures to send out a mailer. I do not think it's a wise investment, so we decided this year for Easter to send a different kind of mail. This [RIP] letter may not go to as many people, but it will have a much greater impact."

> In 2019, churches across the USA donated enough for RIP to abolish $300 million in medical bills.

News of the Dallas campaign spread nationwide within the faith community. RIP soon began hearing from houses of worship across America proposing local debt forgiveness campaigns for their towns and cities. Many miracles.

Fast Forward: In 2019, churches across the USA donated enough funds to help RIP buy and abolish $300 million in hardship medical bills for their communities. Our staff at RIP discovered, regardless of our own beliefs, we'd never before worked with people more sincere and deeply devoted to using medical debt forgiveness for demonstrating unconditional love in the world. Lately, Covid debt is testing our capacity for unconditional love.

Early Medical Debt Summits

Another John Oliver effect has been the series of medical debts summits produced by RIP. Our first summit, held January 2017 in New York City, was created for the university researchers to meet as a team and plan their economic impact study.

This "mini-summit' at the Manhattan office of TheNumber brought together RIP's technology, legal, and data science partners to formulate the practical structure for conducting a randomized controlled trial of medical debt forgiveness.

TransUnion Healthcare agreed to perform data analytics for the study. RIP and TheNumber would handle the debt forgiveness tasks. J-PAL and other benefactors would fund the research. We learned a list of outcomes to be measured was being published in the online research registry of the American Economics Association.

At that summit, Francis Wong cited an Oregon research project that studied the impact of the state's 2008 Medicaid expansion. The findings influenced healthcare policy nationally. Since the medical debt research would have a study group twice the size of the Oregon study, he said, their findings on the impact of medical debt and debt forgiveness might similarly influence public policy.

A hallmark of the annual summits ever since has been a diversity of opinions on the causes of healthcare debt and its possible cures. Our speakers represent health insurance, collections, debt buyers, credit report agencies, health technologists, the Consumer Finance Protection Bureau, Congressional Healthcare Task Force, lobbyists, veterans, economists, and healthcare practitioners.

Summit attendees consistently put aside their job titles, industry loyalties, and agendas to discuss the causes of medical debt and seek pragmatic solutions. Without defending turf, their collegial atmosphere lets everybody listen, speak and be heard with respect.

The most recent 2020 virtual summit focused upon legislation affecting healthcare financing, getting at the root causes of medical debt. Along with discussing the "Medicare for All" proposals being hotly debated in the elections campaigns at the time. We explored the legislative measures in response to the Covid crisis.

All these summit conversations fill me with realistic hope.

The Everyone and Everything Effect

What amazes us daily at RIP is the extent of interest in the relief we provide to people whose debt needs to be forgiven. Attention since John Oliver has often been instigated through media exposure, but we realize that word-of-mouth among caring individuals and organizations is what makes our work possible. Their commitment to forgiving medical debt touches other people's hearts and inspires them to contribute what they can.

We love helping community groups across the United States. They do all of the ground work for putting on their local campaigns. We're honored to be a vehicle for donors to make a concrete difference in the lives of thousands of people in diverse communities. Being in service to these generous souls inspires the RIP staff to feel no less thankful than the recipients of our debt relief.

The vision and mission driving RIP Medical Debt since 2014 is unchanged — locate, buy and abolish medical debt. We had no idea how we would attract the people and funding to make this possible. We simply expected miracles.

Our experience is akin to standing in front of an old-style pinball machine, replete with flashing lights and ringing bells, trying to control a careening silver orb. We've learned a bit about how to use the flippers to direct the ball and hit the bumpers to earn extra turns and enough points to win a free game. Even so, the silver ball of debt forgiveness appears to have a mind of its own, bouncing from pillar to post, lighting up whatever it encounters. It certainly has lit up our future as a charity, perhaps as a movement.

A deeper realization is that RIP and random debt relief cannot ever solve the economic and social problems of medical debt. At best, we can help reduce the heartbreaking, backbreaking burden of medical bills that can never be paid.

We thank John Oliver for initially drawing national attention to the issue of medical debt. We thank all the media bringing public attention to the many social and economic conditions building this mountain of medical debt. We thank all the individuals and community groups now combining forces to stimulate our better angels to influence key people in government and business toward agreeing on humane solutions. Lobbying is how public policy is formulated in the real world. If you happen to be an influencer or "major player," we hope you open a conversation with RIP.

> We can help reduce the heartbreaking, backbreaking burden of medical bills that can never be paid.

The "moral of the story" is that everything that's happened since 2014, everyone who's worked through RIP, has produced the effect of changing our country for the better. People power works.

We've learned to welcome miracles from media and concerned people who get out the story of medical debt and its consequences. All of us are blessed by your own willingness to take action.

"We are the people we've been waiting for."

*Do not accustom yourself to consider
debt only as an inconvenience;
you will find it a calamity.*

— SAMUEL JOHNSON

PART III

Ending
Medical Debt

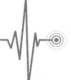

*A hospital bed is a parked taxi
with the meter running.*

— GROUCHO MARX

CHAPTER 10

Health Is a Goal,
Not an Industry

Robert E. Goff

We Americans have an odd concept of healthcare. We will not tolerate people being deprived of it, yet we just don't want to pay for someone else's care. Services essential to a whole community must be paid for by each individual. This results in medical debt for individuals without the resources of insurance or cash.

We debate who should pick up the tab, yet we miss the reality that we *all* pay for the healthcare system. Each of us picks up the tab for the insurance plan premiums, payroll deductions for premiums, deductions for Medicare, taxes for Medicaid, and taxes to subsidize deficits at hospitals and clinics that aren't making it financially. All of us are paying for the losses and consequences of sickness or disability payments, public support of medically indigent families, and economic losses from lost job productivity.

The $3 trillion healthcare spending tab in the USA is about sick care, about accident care, health restoration. It is about the business of providing care, which is not the true business of health.

Shouldn't the discussion about medical debt be much wider? Shouldn't we be as concerned, or far more concerned, about health itself? How can the health status of Americans be lifted? If we'd focus on health not costs, I feel, the costs of care would be positively impacted, stabilized or reduced. Acting to prevent or mitigate illness and injury is not widely perceived as the mission of healthcare. Meanwhile, our health costs keep going up. It defies reason.

Focus on health, not costs. Medical spending should go where it can best improve health.

In my ideal, a health system concerned with patient health would better influence the trajectory of needed care. Utilization of medical services would be decided using a "failure analysis" model to determine the causes of health issues and implement corrective actions. If a patient needs a higher-cost, more intensive care services, that should be taken as a "failure to intervene" earlier with lower-cost, less intensive services. Pay a little now to avoid paying more later.

Too little effort is made to avoid care costs by addressing causes. We know the causes of most illness, but efforts are limited for the interventions that reduce the incidence of illness, reduce costs and improve health outcomes. We know the causes of most injuries, but efforts are limited for the interventions that reduce the incidence of injuries, reduce costs and improve outcomes.

Preventive care helps avoid medical spending. Early intervention forestalls or avoids a costlier intervention later. A healthcare industry paid by delivering care services has no such interest.

The mission and business of the U.S. health industry is treating illnesses and accidents *after* they occur, not before. The industry is compensated for the production and delivery of care services, by service units — a silo of sickness and accident care within the health restoration and repair business.

Medical spending should go where it can best improve health. In the trillions spent annually on medical care, consider the scale of all the missed opportunities. A Kaiser Family Foundation study, for instance, identified factors increasing risks of premature death. Ten percent of premature deaths were due to the care provided. Another 20 percent were due to social or environmental factors, 30 percent to genetics, and 40 percent to personal behaviors.

Health research and treatment has advanced. Illnesses that once meant premature death are now livable chronic conditions, leading to higher levels of medical costs. *Becker's Hospital CFO Report* says unhealthy behaviors are largely responsible for chronic illnesses like heart disease, cancer and diabetes, which pre-Covid caused about 70 percent of all deaths in the USA, and are the most expensive to treat. No one wants to pay for the unhealthy habits of "the other guy."

The Fallacy of Self Reliance

Personal responsibility is an ethical or a moral tenet in America. Freedom entails a natural duty to better oneself responsibly, such as responsibility for one's own health. The ideal of self-reliance explains pushback against national healthcare proposals that reduce personal responsibility. People should face the consequences of their choices. If economic risks from not taking care of oneself are borne by others, in this view, nothing motivates us to engage in healthy behaviors.

Personal responsibility for health is left to individuals. Illness is widely seen as a consequence of poor personal behavior, so prema-ture death is a fitting consequence. I see this as a throwback to the times when poor health signaled a failure in individual piety. The righteous are granted health; the sinful are made to suffer.

By this view, if your behavior increases your risk of illness, if you suffer economic harm as a result, so be it. Equating illness with risky behavior falls apart when that illness is the result of factors outside the control of the individual, such as genetic predispositions, birth defects, environmental factors, or social conditions.

Self-preservation should motivate healthy choices, but we may engage in self-destructive behaviors (like smoking, drinking, drugs) from societal factors (poverty, illiteracy, bigotry). Many causes of illness cannot be addressed by individuals (like pollution). We also cannot yet alter the genetics of our birth.

In the sacred name of personal responsibility or self-reliance, we have shifted the economic cost of health care to patients (like with deductibles and coverage limits). This yields economic hardship for individuals and families, actually making it harder for people to be responsible for themselves.

Self-Destructive Behaviors

Let's look at unhealthy personal behaviors that drive up the costs of healthcare yet begin outside the healthcare system itself.

• *Smoking* — Smoking-related illness costs society more than $300 billion annually, says the Centers for Disease Control (CDC), including $170 billion for direct medical care with $5.6 billion for exposure to secondhand smoke. Taxes on cigarettes to help reduce consumption are offset by manufacturers' discounts to retailers that lower prices for consumers, with about $5.8 billion spent in 2016 to subsidize smoking.

• *Alcohol* — Alcohol abuse costs U.S. society more than $249 billion a year, according to the CDC. Healthcare costs account for only 11 percent of that. A primary cost is lost job productivity.

• *Drug Abuse* — The aggregate cost of drug abuse in the USA is $1 trillion, including costs for medical care and criminal justice. Treasury Secretary Janet Yellen has attributes drug abuse to a lack of job opportunities among prime-age workers. Another vital factor in drug abuse is escape from pain, as with opioid addiction.

• *Gun Violence* — On average, gun misuse costs Americans $700 per person, per year — an annual hit to the economy of $229 billion,

> In the name of personal responsibility, we're making it harder for people to be responsible for themselves.

reports *Mother Jones*. Direct expenses for emergency and medical care from gun violence are $8.6 billion. Wrote doctors in the April 2017 *Annals of Internal Medicine*, "It does not matter whether we believe that guns kill people or that people kill people with guns. The result is the same: A public health crisis."

The Obesity Crisis

America, the "land of plenty," eats ample portion sizes, feeding our waistlines. National Heart, Lung and Blood Institute calculated that since 2000, a bagel grew three inches in diameter to six inches. A cheeseburger grew from 3.5 to 8 ounces. A "normal" serving of sugary soda grew from 6.5 to 20 ounces. The CDC reports almost 40 percent of all U.S. adults and 20 percent of all adolescents are obese. NBC News in 2017 called the obesity crisis "unstoppable."

Obesity is an underlying cause or a contributor to heart disease, stroke, high blood pressure, clots, diabetes, gout, gallbladder disease, osteoarthritis, and such respiratory issues as sleep apnea or asthma.

Obesity is associated with 40 percent of the cancer in the USA. The National Institute of Health cites obesity as a significant risk factor for severe Covid hospitalization and death.

Other nations use taxes on junk food to fight obesity. Taxes on sugary drinks cut soda consumption by 9.7 percent in Mexico. Portugal taxes salt on fattening snacks. Such junk food taxes also exist in Canada, Chile, United Kingdom, Ireland, France, Norway Saudi Arabia, India, South Africa, Thailand, Japan, and Australia. Efforts include banning advertising to children that uses toys as incentives to purchase sugary foods. For behavioral change in the population, these nations aim to change behaviors by increasing the costs at decision-time for such unhealthy behaviors

Other nations use taxes on junk food to fight obesity.

These nations have national health coverage. They use governmental taxing authority to impact behaviors that increase the cost to health care programs. America could learn from them.

In the USA, no national effort exists. We have local initiatives. Philadelphia's tax on sugary drinks shrank soda consumption by 40 percent in 60 days, reported *Philadelphia Magazine*. Energy drink sales fell 64 percent. Bottled water sales rose 58 percent.

The New York Board of Health tried to tax sugary drinks, but an appeals court found the city exceeded its authority. I believe this win for sugary drink producers was a loss for our health.

Embracing the digital life (TV, games, internet) contributes to a sedentary lifestyle, which contributes to obesity. The Robert Wood Johnson Foundation estimated 45 percent of all U.S. adults are not active enough to get daily health benefits. Various diseases related to inactivity cause $117 billion in direct healthcare costs.

Debates over preventative measures for Covid demonstrate the personal responsibility/personal freedom issue. Nothing is clearer than the illness-avoidance value of proven public health measures (masks, immunizations; social distancing), yet common sense met major pushback. Should personal freedom include acceptance of personal and social responsibility? Who decides? Should a Covid patient refusing vaccination forgo care or be charged more for care? Is a refuser responsible for the care costs for all they infect? Should insurance not cover Covid care for vaccine refusers?

Our vaunted healthcare system does little to address unhealthy habits as a source for higher healthcare demand and rising costs. At best, health insurance reimburses a gym membership.

Employers are showing leadership by matching economics with behavior. Some levy higher payroll health insurance deductions for employees who smoke or test with a high Body Mass Index (BMI), a ratio of body fat to height and weight. Some offer employee benefits for gym memberships and usage. Others design office space for more walking around with more stairs to climb. AS for Covid, some controversial employers increase unvaccinated employees' paycheck contributions for health benefits. It's all a start.

Genetics and Health

Genetics powerfully influence our health and longevity. Genes affect 30 percent of our premature deaths. We benefit by knowing in advance our genetic predispositions to diabetes or kidney disease or obesity. We might act to avert illnesses. Early interventions, like a change of diet or monitoring, can make a big difference in not only our own lives but in reducing overall medical care costs.

Genetic testing plays a role in identifying fetuses likely to be born with life-ending, life-threatening birth defects. Amniocentesis, sampling amniotic fluid during pregnancy to screen for fetal abnormalities, is nearly routine. Such testing can detect the likelihood of sickle cell disease, Down syndrome, cystic fibrosis, muscular dystrophy, Tay-Sachs disease, or any diseases where the brain and spinal column do not develop properly, such as spina bifida and anencephaly. How do we act upon that information?

In Iceland, infant Down Syndrome has been virtually eliminated by fetal testing and abortions, reported CBS News *On Assignment.* In developed nations, termination of pregnancies for birth defects is becoming widespread, even in countries with strong anti-abortion cultures, customs and laws.

The Genetic Literacy Project reports genetic testing is becoming part of matchmaking for arranged marriages among Hasidic Jews, who don't sanction abortion. Hasidic high school students get blood drawn for genetic tests. Later, when a match is proposed, the matchmaker and families use the tests to spot risks of genetic diseases or birth defects before they bless or discourage a marriage.

Environmental and Social Factors

Among lower-income groups, a link exists between lower health status and higher health costs. Lack of education limits employment, limiting income, which limits access to quality food, access to healthy working and living conditions, access to quality child care, access to healthcare services, which increases healthcare costs, which increases medical debt, which is a pox upon society.

Nothing in the scope of health insurance can or will address the ecological and social factors contributing to higher health care costs. The healthcare system is not demanding actual upstream solutions. Anti-regulation wave erodes social and environmental protections, yet the impact on healthcare costs should be considered.

The National Environmental Education Foundation reports that more than 1,000 people a day are admitted to hospitals because of chronic lung diseases like asthma, costing the country $56 billion annually in direct care costs (like hospitalization) and indirect costs (missed work and reduced productivity).

Air pollution contributes to 16,000 premature births a year, adding $760 million in direct healthcare costs plus $3.57 billion in lost productivity from physical and mental disabilities, reports *Business Insider*. The Rand Corporation found that in California between 2005 and 2007, air pollution added $193 million in hospital costs, of which Medicare paid $104 million, Medicaid paid $28 million, and private insurances paid the balance of $56 million.

Theory and Reality

Cigna CEO David Cordani told *Business Insider* magazine, "We spend the majority of our money and resources addressing people once they're sick. We need to spend more of our resources keeping people healthy in the first case, and identifying people who are at risk of health events, and lowering those health risks."

No amount of tinkering with insurance models will change that care costs reflect the demand for care and the costs to deliver care. The demand side and structural side create the costs for delivering services. The healthcare industry has been allowed by us to become a voracious monster that threatens to devour every last dollar of America's GDP.

> The healthcare industry has been allowed to become a voracious monster that threatens to devour every last dollar of America's GDP.

Hospitals have emerged as the concentrated economic powers in our healthcare system. They've evolved from local community institutions into networks of care providers composed of urgent care centers (once denigrated as a "doc-in-the-box"), ambulatory surgery centers and the hospital-owned practices and care groups that employ the vast majority of all practicing physicians, says *Becker's Hospital Review*.

> Whether premiums are funded by individual purchases, by employers paying for care benefits, or by taxes, it's all a mechanism for funding the healthcare system.

In theory, such a system could provide great benefits for patients. In-system treatment. theoretically, assures coordination among care-givers, who share patient medical records to avoid costly duplicative testing and conflicting drug inter-actions. In theory, all this lowers the cost of health care by squeezing out unnecessary services within the delivery of care.

An ideal health care structure should lower costs and improve the quality of care. What could be better than this?

Reality is different. All these systems have become additive to higher health care costs rather than reductive. Hospital-dominated systems put the economic needs of the system before the fiscal impact on patients. Revenue is produced by the system and for the system. Efficiencies and economies benefit the system. Patients pay more and more in the process, as do their health insurance companies.

Market Watch tells a tale that is far too common. Jackie Thennes switched to an in-network doctor at a health system facility near her. Her bill suddenly included charges for each doctor visit along with something extra — an added $235 "facility fee."

Concern for maximizing mission has been replaced by concern for maximizing margins.

National Healthcare Policy

All this brings us back to the central problem of medical debt — the proposals, solutions and schemes for who pays and how.

Regardless of your support for or opposition to national health insurance, such as single-payer "Medicare for All," the reality is that the crisis in health insurance coverage and affordability is a crisis in the cost of delivering healthcare. If we bring down the costs of care, we will bring down the volume of medical debt.

Hiding care delivery costs in today's insurance model, or in a nationalized healthcare tax plan, does not change the core structure of care delivery. Neither approach resolves all the factors driving the demand for care. Even if a national health insurance plan is created, high costs for care will still be a major problem.

Opposition to national health insurance, in part, is from a belief the costs will be too great. Given the current trajectory of spending, this objection is valid — up to a point. The Centers for Medicare and Medicaid Services (CMS) projected annual healthcare spending by 2026 will surpass $5.7 trillion dollars. *Investor's Business Daily* says a "Medicare for All" plan would add $32 trillion to federal spending over 10 years, which is $3.2 trillion a year. The current insurance system or a single-payer system will both be expensive.

Health insurance is just a scheme to finance health care services. Whether premiums are funded by individual purchases, by employers paying for care benefits or by taxes, it's just a mechanism for funding the healthcare system to provide care services. Vested interests want to keep the current system in place. Focusing only on insurance misses the demand for services and the many costly way services are delivered. Both must be addressed.

A nation concerned about the quality of its citizens' lives can use taxes to motivate healthier behaviors to reduce a need for care. Tax deductions motivate charity donations to charity. Mortgage deductions motivate home ownership. Taxes on unhealthy behavior shift the cost of care to the pivot point of personal decisions.

It's wrong to make the cost of medical care a barrier to treating the effects of unhealthy behaviors. If costs delay care, it results in still higher costs and poorer outcomes. This is tragic if an illness stems from factors outside a person's control, such as genetic ailments or a respiratory disease caused by secondhand smoke.

The healthcare industry just cannot be expected to reform itself, to be efficient and effective, to find ways of delivering care faster, better and cheaper. It just is not structured to do so. Hospitals, when profitable, do not reduce their costs to the communities that they serve. From noble charities, hospitals have evolved into economic carnivores.

> What matters most in establishing a national healthcare policy is a healthier population, which will reduce the cost of care, and so reduce or eliminate medical debt.

Separate silos for health care delivery, public health and social services do not work. Underfunding public health and social services yields greater demand for healthcare services. Lax environmental quality regulation yields greater demand for care services. Silos raise costs. We need a holistic approach to healthcare costs.

The totality of costs being spent on medical care, public health and social services needs to be considered along with what we know reduces the need for care. Let's allocate services accordingly.

A national healthcare policy needs to be established as a guide. What matters most is a healthier population, which will reduce the cost of care, and so reduce or eliminate medical debt.

A national healthcare policy supports a country that is healthy and an economy that is strong. From such a policy, decisions can be made to support the goal of health, not just care delivery.

A tax policy influencing self-care decisions need not result in a "nanny state" that erodes personal responsibility. Increasing the cost of unhealthy behaviors would deprive no one of the right to engage in such behavior, but would shift the cost to that individual.

Similarly, the cost of pollution needs to shift from the healthcare system to the polluters. Corporations are persons under the law, and should accept personal responsibility for economic freedom.

From a national healthcare policy aimed at improving the health of Americans can flow sensible health benefit plans to promote and support preventative and routine care as well as early interventions for illness along with health maintenance for chronic care.

The structure for delivering care needs to be reconstituted for the betterment of the entire population. A sustainable, affordable funding model then becomes a possibility, be it insurance, Medicare for All, or some other national health plan.

The present system is rigged against citizen health. This is done not by design or a cabal of evil doers, but by the historical evolution of our healthcare delivery structure. We need an evolution to higher thinking for the health of everyone in America.

Covid overlaid the issues of personal responsibility and public policy. Political perspectives in the communal environment resulted in science and facts being subject to ideology. Unlike in the 14th century Black Death pandemic, when Europeans put all their faith in flower garlands, today we know bubonic plague does not come "bad air" but from bacteria carried by fleas. In 21st century America, our yearnings for individual freedom collide with science-based public health realities like masks and vaccinations.

> We need an evolution to higher thinking for the health of everyone in America.

Our modern pandemic has shown society is prepared to accept the cost of communal medical care regardless of the ability to pay. Emergency bipartisan legislation funded community hospitals and opened temporary emergency hospitals, such as converting parking garages into treatment centers, developing and distributing "free" vaccines to anyone, regardless of party affiliation.

However, the politics of the crisis did not translate into rational public policy. Refusals to adhere to public health recommendations and rules, plus premature curtailment of public health restrictions, have yielded higher illness rates and death tolls, which all was avoidable. Dismissing the adage that "an ounce of prevention is worth a pound of cure," politicizing the pandemic produced higher levels of healthcare costs and lower levels of overall health. Such a disconnect is not sensible, nor sustainable. To paraphrase the famous old Pogo comic strip, "We have met the problem, and it is us."

I believe we can do better.

CHAPTER 11

Personal and Societal Medical Debt Solutions

Craig Antico

Every day I see our healthcare system causing financial ruin for millions of Americans, their friends and families. Many of them would be financially ruined no matter what they do or we do. That's unacceptable. This chapter can help assure such ruin does not happen to you or those you love. I also will speak here about systemic things we can do as a country to avoid these horrid outcomes.

Until then, let's get personal. Illnesses, accidents or attacks often cause unexpected shocks. Material hardships often ensue. There are useful steps you can take — or your friends and family can take — that are in your personal control. Such actions can help you mitigate the risk of the medical debt hardship.

Nothing is sadder to me than seeing people make poor decisions about their own health care and wellness because of ignorance or an unwillingness to act. Nothing makes me angrier than the number of people in positions of authority who are unwilling to educate and support people in need, so they can help themselves.

There is no other nation in the world like the United States that tries as hard as we do to make up for systemic disparities, inequalities and government inefficiencies. Nor is there another land that freely donates more time and money for the good of other people. When Americans become aware of others' unmet need, like after a wildfire or hurricane, we do our best both as givers and as recipients of giving. This fact gives me hope.

Personal Responsibility Solutions

Many of us are just one illness or accident away from financial ruin or material hardship from medical debt. Hardship can occur for you and others when you or any person...

1. Ignores health care billing notices.
2. Doesn't have or take the time to stay current on their bills.
3. Doesn't read through the medical bills they get.
4. Waits until they're in a crisis to act.
5. Asks you or another to pay any bill for them.
6. Puts bills on a credit card (worse if you co-signed).
7. Doesn't feel the need to have any health insurance.

When it comes to material hardship, I've seen it all in my work. As one whose family has experienced material hardship, I wish to help you to avoid or mitigate such deep scars by teaching you how to take better personal responsibility for your own health care costs. Doing your own part inspires others to do theirs. From our sense of personal responsibility will flow greater social responsibility.

If you have everything under full control, and you're properly insured, you can ignore the tips below. These are tips I've garnered in the 30 years that I've been in this business of cleaning up the debt mess created by our healthcare system. I've also learned what to do from my own hardship. These actions can be helpful.

Below is a self-help guide with basic how-to information.

For Individual Patients

• *Stay Healthy and Safe* — Help protect yourself from medical bills through wellness and fitness practices. As much as possible in your life, sensibly practice precautions to avoid injury or infection or exposure to violence.

• *Are you Underinsured or Uninsured?* — Your health policy's deductible should not exceed five percent of your gross income. If your deductible is higher, you are underinsured. Any illness or injury could cause financial hardship that endures for years.

The cheapest health insurance likely is no bargain. If you earn less than two times the Federal Poverty Level (FPL), your deductible should not pass five percent of your gross income. If you earn more, your deductible should not pass 10 per cent of your gross income. If you earn $30,000, the deductible should be no more than $1,500 a year. If you earn near $60,000, the deductible cap should be $6,000 a year. This is a rule of thumb.

> Your policy's deductible should not exceed 5% of your gross income. If your deductible is higher, you are underinsured.

If your deductible is any higher than the above guidelines, your family is underinsured. If you have one major illness or accident, you and your family are vulnerable to material hardship that could last from three to five years.

If you can't pay for insurance, the Affordable Care Act's subsidy Marketplace may help. If you can't afford even this, be sure to ask if you qualify for Medicaid. You also may qualify for charity care.

• *Understand Your Health Insurance* — The Commonwealth Fund finds that 68 million people in America are underinsured or uninsured; these people often have medical debt. To protect yourself, research how health insurance works and doesn't work (reread this book). Understand such key concepts as co-insurance, co-payments, deductibles, in-network, and out-of-network benefits.

Before you need care, find out which care providers are and are not covered by your own in-network plan.

If you are insured, be clear exactly what your plan covers. Be clear about your insurance policy' terms and conditions. Study the sections about co-insurance, co-payments, deductibles, and out-of-network costs. Read all the fine print. Be a conscious healthcare consumer.

Figure that 25 to 30 percent of all your healthcare costs will come out of your own pocket in the form of deductibles, co-pays and co-insurance premiums.

• *Identify All Your In-Network Providers* — Before you need care, find out which care providers are and are not covered by your in-network plan. A hospital may be in-network, but providers there may not, such as the ambulance, emergency room, radiologists, and clinical laboratories.

If you live in a region with only one hospital, you are at high risk of not having many or any in-network doctors nearby. However, this can happen in any hospital anywhere that participates in only a few insurance plans, even in urban areas.

Above all, find out in advance of a medical crisis whether your local ambulance company and hospital emergency room staff is in-network. They may not be. They most probably are out-of-network contractors, so you could get a bill five to ten times the cost of in-network charges for the same care services.

• *Pin Down your Care Charges in Advance* — As much as possible, get care providers to specify in advance of any visit and procedure or visit what they will do, what they will charge, and if your insurance covers it. The goal is avoiding surprise charges.

Along with ensuring all providers are in network, as much as feasible, pin down the exact dollar amounts for expected charges. Always get written estimates when exact charges cannot be nailed down, as with major surgery. Adria Gross from MedWise Insurance Advocacy warns, "Whatever agreed fee amount you have with your medical provider, make sure you have it in writing."

• *Know Your 'Balance Billing' Consumer Rights* — The practice of billing a patient for whatever insurance does not cover is called "balance billing." The practice puts the patient at risk of a surprise medical bill for the unpaid balance.

A *New England Journal of Medicine* study in 2016 found that 22 percent of emergency room visits nationally involved care by an out-of-network doctor. Almost a quarter of ER visits produced bills that could become personal medical debt.

A 2018 Yale study found out-of-network billing was concentrated into a relatively small number of hospitals. They found that 50 percent of hospitals have out-of-network billing below two percent of the total billing, while 15 percent of hospitals have out-of-network billing rates above 80 percent.

Study author Zack Cooper, assistant professor of health policy and economics at Yale University, told Kellie Schmitt of the USC Annenberg Center for Health Journalism, "These sorts of surprise bills can tally up into the hundreds or thousands of dollars, and really wreak financial havoc on people's lives."

The practice of "balance billing" is prohibited for patients on Medicaid or Medicare. A hospital agrees to accept what the government pays for a care service, waiving any further amounts.

New Jersey in 2018 enacted law against balance billing, described by the Governor, Phil Murphy, as "one of the strongest consumer protection laws in the country." At the signing ceremony, he said an estimated 168,000 patients in New Jersey get out-of-network bills that total $420 million annually, adding $1 billion annually to health costs. Other states have proposed or enacted similar laws, but no national balance billing law exists.

So, as a personal policy, always ask if your care providers are in-network. Failure to ask could mean medical debt.

• *Examine Bills Carefully* — Adria Gross says that "about eighty percent of all medical bills have errors." The procedure code, for instance, may contain an error from an overwhelmed staffer doing hasty keyboard input. Billing errors also could be systemic, invisible to the provider, unknown to the software developer. You would do everyone a favor by questioning every billing code. Errors rarely are deliberate, so be gracious when reporting an issue.

With a bit of practice, you can learn how to spot billing errors when you see them. The learning curve is rewarding.

First, always insist upon receiving an itemized bill rather than a summary statement. Undertake an internet search for the meaning of each procedure code itemized. Once you understand the codes, ask yourself, are any procedures inexplicable, don't make sense, or don't fit what you recall happening? Make notes about all the codes inviting inquiry. Also notate the codes appearing often, even if due and proper, for there may be limits on what insurance will cover.

Look up each procedure code on a bill. Research the "reasonable and customary charges" for that code. Compare the usual charge for that code to the charge on your bill. If there is any mismatch, you have good cause to contact your health providers with an inquiry or challenge. Being polite and friendly will help you get positive results. Anger provokes resistance.

Wait 30-45 days before calling. Miscoding mistakes on bills often take three months for insurance billing departments to process.

If on Medicare, carefully review your quarterly Summary Notice. Check the codes to see if you spot any errors. For any procedures Medicare declines to cover, contact your care provider in case they can fix a coding error and resubmit a charge. You also may appeal any declined charge to Medicare. Find the appeal process in any quarterly statement with a denial.

• *Beware of Facility Fees* — Hospital-owned physician practices often charge "facilities fees" above the usual service charge. A facility fees can occur if the doctor is described as "affiliated" with a

> Look up each procedure code on a bill. Research the 'reasonable and customary charges' for that code. Compare the usual charge for that code to the charge on your bill.

hospital. In Washington State, for instance, a patient paid $125 out-of-pocket to visit a hospital-employed doctor, but charges for the visit soared to more than $500 to reflect a new facility fee.

The Physician Advocacy Institute asserts facility fees are being charged much more than before because hospitals now own about 30 percent of physician practices and employ over 70 percent of all the practicing physicians in our nation.

Hospitals and medical practices have the legal right to charge facilities fees, even where a physician's office is off-campus from the hospital. The problem is most visible when patients go to the same place they've always gone for care services, and they don't expect to get charged more.

Ask in advance if there will be a facility fee. If there will be, ask if your procedure can be done at a facility that doesn't charge such a fee.

So, whenever possible, before you incur medical bills from any hospital-owned practices, always ask in advance of a visit if you will be charged a facility fee. Bear in mind that facility fees may apply to any office, on and off a hospital campus, or when a doctor is only "affiliated" with a hospital.

Always ask in advance if there will be a facility fee. If there will be, ask if your procedure can be done at a facility that does not charge such a fee. Fighting the fee afterwards is close to impossible.

• *Only Visit the ER in a Genuine Emergency* — Call your doctor if an issue is not life-threatening. Go to the emergency room only if your doctor says to go. To help avoid issues with your insurance, document the doctor's office advice or referral to visit the ER. (My spouse did make that call, but she was in excruciating pain and later could not remember who said to go to the ER. We had to pay a $700 ER bill that could have been a $150 co-pay.)

Take good notes. Record the day, exact time, and name of the person who told you to go (check spelling). Insist upon a notation in your records that your condition warranted an ER visit.

• *Always File Out-of-Network Claims* — Insurance companies can process and pay your out-of-network ("OON") bill as much as seven years after the OON bill was generated. So, always submit out-of-network charges to your insurance company.

You can be reimbursed after a bill was paid by you, by friends or by family. About $55 billion each year is given by friends and family for medical expenses and debt repayment. If you do not file a claim for your own benefit, do it to repay your friends and family.

Do not ask your doctor or hospital to file the OON claim for you. It's not in their interest to do so. They have already been paid. Why would they help you get reimbursed?

Given more than $400 billion a year being billed OON, and an accumulated trillion in out-of-network debt left unpaid over the last ten years, there's a potential for us to recover $40 million dollars from insurance companies. So, get OON it!

• *Do Not Pay with Credit Cards or Interest-Bearing Loans* — Never pay medical bills with high-interest credit cards or payday loans. Unless repaid quickly, such financial instruments may cost you double the actual debt. Instead, negotiate an interest-free installment payment agreement with your medical provider. No credit is needed for it, and it will not show on your credit report if you ever miss a payment, providing you catch up quickly.

The main way medical debt from a hospital or doctor becomes an interest-bearing "debt" is when you ignore it, get sued, ignore that or lose the case, and find a judgment entered against you. Your risk is compounded if you forestall a suit by paying with a card or loan.

If you have debt at a high-interest rate, such as a credit card or a payday loan, you can help yourself by researching the "Rule of 76" and the higher interest "Rule of 78." Low-interest loans, like home equity loans, use the "Rule of 72." Understanding these rules may spare you from real hardship.

The Rule of 76 calculates how soon the amount you owe will double. To do it, divide 76 by your interest rate, let's say 24 percent. Working the formula: 76 ÷ 24% = 3.17 years to double what you owe. The Rule of 76 tells you that the $3,000 you put on a credit card turns into $6,000 in about three years! Ouch!

If possible, refinance high-interest credit card debt to get a lower interest rate. If you must leverage collateral, like with a car or house, be certain you can and will meet the terms of the obligation.

Whenever possible, make an interest-free installment payment agreement with the medical provider. You may be surprised at how willing they are to work with you, since so few patients know to ask for a payment plan. Being honest with them, letting them see you are being responsible, may yield unexpected benefits.

• *Always Pay On-Time* — Whenever you make an agreement with a creditor to pay any medical bill, do all in your power to make all agreed payments when due, or before. Missed and late payments ding your credit rating, and if chronic can cripple your finances.

Sustained on-time payments tend to uplift your credit rating, which benefits your ability to secure vehicles, housing and jobs.

• *Communicate with Providers and Collectors* — If paying a bill will cause hardship for you or your family, tell your hospital or bill collector. Answer all their calls. Explain the situation. Be honest and realistic. They may actually help you.

If you are going to miss a payment for any reason, inform the creditor immediately. If you have any change in your circumstances that adversely affects your ability to pay on time, like a job loss or illness, inform the creditor promptly. Because so few people exhibit such personal responsibility, the creditor very likely will be willing to adjust your arrangements. Ask about changing the due date or the amount being paid, even if short-term. They probably will be thrilled you want to pay anything at all.

• *Start or Max-Out Your Health Savings Account* — Save money for future medical expenses in a federally insured, tax-free account to use as you wish for self-pay medical care, like diagnostic testing. You own and control all the money in your HSA, not your employer or insurer. Fund the maximum annual contribution to an HSA, which can pay for itself.

A 2017 Kaiser Family Foundation survey found 46 percent of those in high-deductible health plans reported difficulty affording deductibles. About 60 percent with employer-sponsored health insurance have high deductible passing $1,300 for an individual and $2,750 for a family. An HSA fosters resiliency and helps avert medical debt. Try to fund the maximum annual contribution in your HSA.

> An HSA has a significant tax benefit. You don't pay taxes on the money put into the plan, nor do you pay taxes on the amount you spend on your medical expenses or premiums.

An HSA has a significant tax benefit. You don't pay taxes on the money put into the plan, nor do you pay taxes on the amount you spend on your medical expenses or insurance premiums. IRS rules for 2021 let you contribute up to $3,600 per year as an individual, or $7,200 for a family. The IRS allows a catch-up contribution up to $1,000 a year for people age 55 or over.

Once you're on Medicare at age 65, you can't contribute to an HSA, so if you're younger, start an HSA now. Stop funding your HSA six months before you join Medicare to avoid any IRS issues.

• *Pay only Three to Six Percent of Your Gross Income on Out-of-Pocket Expenses or Medical Debt* — Hardship can occur when medical expenses reach as little as two percent of your gross income. Research shows most people experience hardship when their out-of-pocket (OOP) expenses rise above 2.5 percent of gross income.

You may have more resiliency than others. Only you know how much you can afford to pay in a given year for OOP expenses and past debt. Your savings, a second job, or family and friends can help mitigate hardship, which fosters resiliency, reduces your stress and enhances your health.

> Most people experience hardship when their out-of-pocket medical expenses rise above 2.5% of gross income.

To stay within that three to six percent of your gross income for OOP expenses, if possible, make a yearly projection for six percent of your annual gross income. Within that budget, only pay out what you can afford. If any account is in collections, pay only what you can afford. Even if you get collection calls, be resolute that you will not stop taking your medications, going to the doctor, paying rent and utilities, or putting tires on your car for safely going to a job. No one can force you to pay a bill instead of life necessities. You alone always control whom to pay and how much you pay.

• *Determine Eligibility for Charity Care Before You Need It* — If you are in hardship, in advance of receiving hospital care, if you can, research the websites of local providers for their "charity care policy" or "financial assistance policy." Hospitals are required to post this policy publicly, but you may need to search the site to find it.

Most hospitals offer free charity care for low income patients. To qualify, generally, your income must be below 200 percent of the Federal Poverty Level, two times the FPL. If you earn above that, the hospital may have a sliding scale for bill payment, from 10 percent to 80 percent of the total bill. (You can find online Federal Poverty Level guidelines and calculators at HealthCare.gov.)

You may qualify for free medical care, or fees on a sliding scale, but you must ask! Hospitals rarely offer free or lower-fee care on their own. Crucially, you must ask for charity care when admitted. Once admitted as a "self-pay" patient, the hospital expects to be paid in full. One-third of all hospital accounts in collections qualified for charity care, but patients did not get it or know to ask for it.

Physicians practicing independent of hospitals, as a rule, do not offer charity care, except in rare cases, for they cannot afford to do so, and keep their doors open. I bless doctors who volunteer for charity clinics in underserved communities, who work there, or create such clinics. Every year on average, we Americans personally give away to charity about two percent of our gross domestic product (GDP). Some may wish to see our generosity grow.

What's stunning to me is that 33 percent of the U.S. population earns less than two times the FPL (about $40,000 to $50,000), and the low earners are the most generous givers to charity, as well as needy friends and family (F&F). As a percentage of adjusted gross income, this segment gives away far more than those in much higher income brackets. Lower-income people give more, even if it brings hardship, because they know first-hand what a big difference generosity makes in their own lives and other people's lives.

• *Apply for Medicaid in Case of Low Income* — Poverty may last a lifetime and endure endemic for generations. Low income, by itself often is a temporary situation. I'm talking from experience. U.S. law offers a remedy for both.

Medicaid is the health insurance for all low-income citizens who can't afford their medical care expenses. Income qualification criteria vary state-to-state, so contact your state Medicaid office to see if you qualify. Your child may be eligible for Medicaid even if you are not. Learn the eligibility rules for the state where you live.

If you qualify, Medicaid will pay all approved care if you stay in-network. People on Medicaid incur no medical debt. Medicaid may pay recently medical bills, too, but only within a short timeframe, like 90 to 180 days. If you may qualify for Medicaid, even if temporarily, apply very soon after receiving an unpayable care bill.

If you are up to age 26 and on your parent's insurance, consider applying for Medicaid. We don't know anybody on Medicaid with medical debt problems, including recent graduates looking for a job. Consider yourself fortunate if you have parental plan coverage, yet they'll consider themselves as fortunate if you have a major illness or injury, when your Medicaid spares them from financial ruin.

• *Sign up for Medicare When Qualified* — Apply for Medicare as soon as you are eligible at age 65 (under current law). The Forbes Finance Council warns of significant penalties for late enrollment into Medicare. These penalties accumulate the longer you wait to enroll, and they can be costly.

To be precise, pending Congressional actions, you have a seven-month enrollment period starting three months before and after the month you turn 65. Enroll in Medicare Parts A, B and D during this period if you don't have better health coverage.

Medicare only covers 80 percent of an authorized charge. That unpaid 20 percent could become medical debt. So, if you can afford a Medicare supplemental plan, buy one. "Medigap" insurance covering that 20 percent gap could mean the difference between solvency and hardship if you get sick or injured. Find the most comprehensive supplemental plan you can afford.

Do all your homework before making decisions on your Medicare parts, like a third-party prescription Part D plan. Investigate the diverse supplemental plans. Compare premium rates. Check out consumer reviews and complaints. Be careful.

You can instead buy a Medicare replacement "Medicare Advantage" plan,. Private insurance companies contract with Medicare to provide Medicare Part A and B benefits. Your insurer becomes this private company, not the U.S. government. Some critics call Advantage plans a disadvantage, mainly in the case of coverage disputes or slow payments to providers. As with the Medigap supplemental plans, carefully do all your homework before you buy any Advantage plan. Check reviews and consider complaints.

Even with Medicare, according to a Fidelity analysis, a 65-year-old couple that retires today could need $280,000 to cover all their expected combined care costs before death. Good supplemental coverage is one of the most important things you can do to limit or avoid medical debt during retirement.

Do all your homework before making decisions on your Medicare parts, like a third-party prescription Part D plan. Investigate the diverse supplemental Medigap plans. Compare plan premium rates. Check out consumer reviews and complaints. Be careful.

For Caregivers

With more than 25 million seniors living below 250 percent of the FPL, more caregivers are needed, and families can't cope. If you are one of the 35 million adult children caring for a parent, or you're one of the 15 million caring for a spouse, or one of 35 million parents taking care of adult children with disabilities, you are keenly aware of the costs involved in caregiving.

The average paid by families for OOP expenses per year is more than $,7000, but figure in lost wages for caregivers, added stress, and the other hidden costs. About 48 million family caregivers annually provide $470 billion in unpaid care. If you're a caregiver, your gift of love should not harm you.

Here are things you can do as a caregiver to help yourself:

• *Claim Due Income Tax Deductions* — If you meet the IRS requirements, if you care for an aging parent in your home, you may qualify to file as the head of household. If you pay a parent's medical expenses that are not reimbursed by insurance, if you itemize, you might claim a deduction.

• *Get The Caregiving Tax Credit* — Those providing care for a family member can get a tax credit under the Credit for Caring Act. Eligible family caregivers can get a credit for 30 percent of qualified expenses above $2,000 paid OOP to help a loved one. The maximum tax credit amount is $3,000. The Credit for Caring Act of 2021 may raise this to $5,000, if enacted.

• *Use Medicaid-Paid Caregiving Programs* — Medicaid in your state may offer a way to get paid for taking care of a family member, friend or neighbor. New York State, for instance, has the Consumer Directed Personal Assistance Program (CD-PAP), a Medicaid-funded program that helps care recipients hire almost any caregiver they wish, including the family member providing care. Freedom Care NY provides services statewide.

According to Medicaid market analyst Athena Mandros, most state Medicaid programs offer some form of self-directed care, which is used by more than 800,000 people nationwide. Your state also may offer ways to pay you for taking care of a family member, friend or neighbor. Ask your local Medicaid office.

• *Be a Compensated Caregiver* — Beyond Medicaid, programs and mechanisms exist to ease the expense and lost income for a family caregiver. Long-term care insurance as well as worker compensation insurance may pay for your family members to be caregivers.

You also can draft an "eldercare contract" among family members that outlines care duties and provides a way to pay the caregiver. For help, The National Academy of Elder Law Attorneys assists seniors with legal issues and people of all ages with disabilities. They can help you draft an eldercare contract to end all the confusion among family members. Be sure the caregiver has a voice in drafting this contract.

> Draft an 'eldercare contract' among family members that outlines care duties and a way to pay the caregiver.

An eldercare agreement lets the family pool resources to pay for a caregiver when the care recipient lacks means. If a care recipient has ample resources, an agreement can avoid or mitigate feuds between family members on who inherits money or gifts. It further can ensure the caregiver is treated with deserved respect, especially if a caregiver must stop working to help the loved one.

For veterans, the VA may honor an OOP caregiving claim if the care receiver is a vet. The VA also may provide home care services in your community. If your loved one is a veteran, contact the Veteran Directed Home and Community-Based Services (VDHCBS), which pays vet family members to act as caregivers.

The above tips are by no means comprehensive, but if you apply them, you may spare yourself from hardship due to medical debt.

General Systemic Solutions

Even without a pandemic, as personal income grows at a slower rate, as predicted, the cost of health care is expected to double in the next seven to ten years. Government now pays 70 percent of these costs. No matter who pays a medical bill, it will be impossible to pay for all care without a revolution in cost reductions, backed by more effective care delivery and greater personal wellness.

Increasing the emphasis upon wellness in society will reduce the health care costs trajectory, and so help end medical debt. In lieu of major new laws that alter the U.S. healthcare system, we can make a major impact on reducing medical debt through these strategies:

Make Charity Care and Medicaid 'Opt-Out'

More than a third of all medical debt comes from care services provided by nonprofit hospitals. A simple solution for part of our medical debt epidemic would be to make charity care and Medicaid *opt-out*. Those who quality under the hospital's financial assistance policy (FAP) would automatically get needed care for free. Patients could decline or opt-out of free care, but I expect few would.

To qualify for charity care today, hospitals require patients to provide extensive verification of income, assets or hardship. The onus has been upon the patients, so too few ever apply, even if they know free or reduced-cost charity care is available.

RIP can provide to hospitals the data and analytics to connect their clinical data with federal Health and Human Services networks to verify patients' eligibility for charity care. This innovative link between a Health Information Exchange (HIE) and a Community Information Exchange (CIE) shows great promise for identifying patients qualified for charity care. With RIP involved, we can cancel medical debt on the spot.

As our proof-of-concept, RIP engaged in a first-of-its-kind pilot with "211 San Diego," the social service resource and information hub. Using their CIE, we connected two participating hospitals with 6,000 health and human services providers in San Diego to identify charity care cases and to abolish medical debt for qualified patients. The initial pilot project suggests the possibilities.

Imagine charity care, Medicaid enrollment and debt cancellation for eligible people being automatic, so patients in hardship would have to consciously, deliberately opt-out to avoid the benefit.

> It will be impossible to pay for all care without a revolution in cost reductions, backed by more effective care delivery and greater personal wellness.

Build 'Data Trusts,' so Consumers Control Their own Data

Health care services, like all ventures, spend money for personal data to identify who needs their services, and they expend revenue improving their services to make them more attractive.

Personal data about our wellness, finances and consumer behavior should be private. Lack of data privacy breeds social distrust.

> I envision 'data trusts' where patients and consumers own, control and monitor their private personal data, which legally belongs to them, not to corporations or the state.

Products and services could be ethically based on reliable medical data systems that patients control themselves. Care services could be delivered in real time using secure fully anonymized data on patients, families, and communities. If care provider decisions are driven by data-informed evidence, this could lower costs across every healthcare sector, reducing medical debt.

To accomplish this, I support using a data flow science pioneered over two decades by OBASHI in Scotland, deployed internationally. I envision "data trusts" where all patients and consumers own, control and monitor their private personal data, which legally belongs to them, not to corporations or the state. Privacy protections in secure data trusts would strengthen the protections in the Health Insurance Portability and Accountability Act (HIPAA).

Let Specialty Finance Companies Abolish Medical Debt

Hospitals and doctors are getting out of the business of letting you owe them money, collecting bills and incurring bad debt. They want immediate payment. Some don't participate in insurance plans, government or private. They take only cash or credit cards.

Some hospitals or doctors assign their billing to a bank specialty finance company, such as CareCredit. In these instances, you may owe a bank for your care without ever knowing it, never realizing you don't owe anything directly to the hospital or doctor.

In my mind, this trend could be harmful to patients financially. To offset the risks of medical debt owed to banks rather than to care providers, I propose that these specialty finance companies establish a fund to forgive the medical debt of those in hardship. Such a fund could be created by any company or the specialty finance industry acting in unison. This could become a nationwide practice.

Build a Charity Fund to Pay Caregivers for Caregiving

Helpful caregivers are burdened by medical debt due to giving care. Caregiving more and more causes hardship for our dwindling caregiver base. We need a good safety net for them. We need more education on the programs out there for caregivers. Caregiving itself needs to be better funded. I propose we unite to establish state and national charitable funds for this purpose.

About $400 billion in caregiving services are rendered each year, and much of that is lost income. This is the same amount as the $400 billion that citizens, corporations and foundations give to charities every year. Caregivers rarely get trained in the fiscal matters affecting them. Few are aware some states and organizations actually pay for caregivers. We can do more to support them as a society.

Shift Who Pays for Severely Past Due, Unpayable Debt

I've run debt collection companies all of my adult life. Before founding RIP with Jerry Ashton, also a debt collections veteran, we worked in an industry that earned $19 billion a year in revenue, half of that from medical debt collections, $6 billion in debt settlement and debt consolidation, and another $5 billion from credit repair. The industry also earned $50 billion from debt settlements collected for creditor clients. That's a fast profile of the industry.

I estimate 20 to 25 percent of all the debtors were in hardship at the time they paid their debts. If we educated those in hardship to safely, privately self-identify their hardship, our communities could pay their debts for them through charitable debt buying and abolishment, as RIP does. If we'd share the debt burden, we'd cut material hardship to practically nothing.

> A shift of just $2 billion in our national wealth to buy and forgive older medical debt could eradicate all the medical debt hardship in America.

A shift of just $2 billion in our national wealth to buy older medical debt (at a penny on the dollar) can abolish $200 billion in medical debt and eradicate all the medical debt hardship in America. Such national medical debt forgiveness is possible with enough donations by those without debt, or with debt who can afford to donate.

Given a trillion in unpayable healthcare bills in America over the past decade, such a small shift in our national wealth can make a large dent in U.S. medical debt. If we reduce this pressure on our economy, we may find more permanent answers for finally ending medical debt, such as by increasing wellness, by reducing costs, and by changing how we finance care delivery in our nation.

CHAPTER 12

National Health Care:
To Be or Not To Be?

Jerry Ashton

W e're living in a particularly hard time for American society. There's wide agreement our healthcare system is broken, but when it comes to repairing it, forget about any reasoned discourse. You're damned if you pick any side, such as for or against single-payer, and you are damned no matter which side you pick. If you try to say neutral, you're condemned by all sides.

Fixed positions on healthcare are now expected for members of every social group, economic class, religion, or political persuasion. Justifications for a strident position will and must be found. Minds are closed. Why argue? Give up and move on.

Meanwhile, our broken healthcare system screams for change. It's equivalent to "global warming" in healthcare economics. Every degree that care costs rise creates a hotter and costlier future. As in climate change, deniers refuse to admit our care structure ensures medical debt will keep rising until we change our ways.

Our society is now as fractured as our healthcare system. Each proposed "solution" is opposed, often by the same interests creating the problem. Some feel locked into the current system by a career or paycheck. Others are locked into a political or religious ideology that defines what's right and wrong. The refusal to compromise is a righteous moral stand, and all doubts are treason.

What stances are we willing to give up to make healthcare work? What are we willing to do to make America healthier, equitable and fully sustainable? No matter what solution we may pick, implementation will not be easy, and it will not be perfect.

> No matter what solution we may pick, implementation will not be easy, and it will not be perfect.

Is medical debt forgiveness the solution? Well, yes and no. Yes, because cancelling unpayable bills surely helps the beneficiaries of debt relief. No, because medical debt forgiveness treats symptoms but does not cure the disease.

The sources of medical debt reside "upstream" in social determinants. Until those factors change, righting a wrong by forgiving debt, however sincere and well-intended, will not permanently rid America of medical debt. Given at least $1 trillion of medical debt over the past ten years, given $40 billion currently, even if RIP keeps growing and abolishes two or three billion dollars in medical debt a year, that will do almost nothing to change the existing healthcare system. Debt forgiveness, by itself, can never make a real dent in all the debt that's been created, is now being created and will be created tomorrow. We need fundamental changes in the healthcare system's structure and economics.

The good news is that RIP and our allies are calling attention to the problem of medical debt and facilitating the process of finding solutions that work. As a tax-exempt charitable organization under U.S. law, we must remain nonpartisan. Still, we can join with people and organizations engaged in the monumental efforts to inform and change public opinion — change public policy. Our collective voices and actions finally can end medical debt.

Ideally, we'd love to see our charity put out of business. No medical debt would mean no need to forgive it. Ending medical debt for all can happen once Americans agree we need radical changes in the financial structure for delivering medical care.

The tide is turning. I see Americans removing their blinders and challenging the status quo, honestly looking at bold alternatives and innovations. We are recognizing with empathy that not only are we "our brother's keeper," we all are one family.

This chapter looks at the main proposals to create such positive changes in our healthcare system.

A Modern Barn Raising

Traditionally in our country, if a rural family's livelihood was ruined by a major financial loss, like a barn destroyed by a fire or tornado, the community would show up and pitch in, unpaid, to build a replacement barn. Some contributed labor, some lumber or nails, others money, but all contributed from their hearts.

There was enlightened self-interest in those community efforts. People knew, "It could be me someday," so everybody pitched in vigorously, even joyfully (as in Habitat for Humanity). People knew that if disaster struck in their own lives, their friends, neighbors and relatives would return the social investment.

Today, for the donors and friends of RIP Medical Debt, perhaps unconsciously, we serve a similar role for social investment. Many of our donors sense, at some level, that medical debt — a bad credit report, bankruptcy, job loss, the inability to finance a car, rent an apartment or buy a house — could well be in their future. We accept that our own "barn" may need raising someday.

If nothing changes in healthcare financing, none of us are safe from unexpected, catastrophic medical bills. Your family, social rank or education will not save you.

> If nothing changes in healthcare financing, none of us are safe from catastrophic medical bills.

Consider the case of a Nobel Prize-winning physicist, Leon Lederman, dying in 2018 at age 96. His wife told Associated Press for his obituary that in 2015 he'd sold his Nobel Prize medallion at auction for $765,000 "to help pay for medical bills and care." If you know anyone hit by medical bills for Covid, you must realize that no one is invulnerable.

In the spirit of civic education and open discourse, let's look at four of the most widely supported solutions now being proposed for fixing U.S. healthcare:

1. Improve the Affordable Care Act.
2. Regulate insurance and drug prices.
3. Public option and Medicare expansion.
4. Medicare for All, single-payer healthcare

A *caveat*: What follows is not comprehensive, nor is it meant to be, but this is enough to help you think reasonably and realistically about these main four options. The goal is raising awareness. What you do with that awareness — such as seeking more education or becoming more actively involved — is up to you.

Improve the Affordable Care Act

The battle cry of "Repeal and Replace" fell silent in response to voter outrage in the 2018 mid-term elections, rejecting politicians who would stop coverage for preexisting conditions and ending the "individual mandate" that every American has health insurance.

Writer John Hecht wrote for *Bustle* an insightful article, "Repeal and Replace is Dead," He tracked the Republican efforts to kill "Obamacare" and gave reasons for their failure. The chief reason for failure was that "Republican lawmakers couldn't quite stomach it." Defunding the ACA would drive up health insurance premiums to stratospheric levels. Repealing the ACA subsidies would then cause 32 million voters to lose their insurance. Further chilling GOP ardor was their pummeling at town halls by angry constituents, who in 2018 voted many of them out of office.

A group of senators and representatives cobbled-together a "skinny bill" that failed to win enough votes. A silent thumbs-down by Sen. John McCain (R-AZ) hammered the stake through the heart of his party's sole viable offering.

Sen. Lindsey Graham(R-SC) summed up the GOP's seven years fight to repeal and replace the ACA. "I thought everybody else knew what the hell they were talking about, but apparently not."

Undeterred, the GOP-controlled Congress and conservative-leaning Supreme Court undercut the fines upholding the individual mandate. This ruling provided a basis for Republican state attorneys general to file a lawsuit against the ACA. The Trump administration did not defend the hated Obamacare. A federal district court judge in Texas, ignoring the principle of severability, ruled in late 2018 that the entire ACA is unconstitutional.

A group of states governed by Democrats appealed the ruling, and as the case wound its way back to the Supreme Court, the ACA remained in effect. Those 133 million Americans with preexisting conditions remained protected under the ACA. The 20 million Americans relying on the ACA for their health insurance remained covered. In June 2021, the Supreme Court again ruled the individual mandate to have health insurance is constitutional, which put an end to all calls to "repeal and replace" the ACA, not that Republicans ever actually offered a comprehensive replacement plan.

Later, in response to Covid, the 2020 CARES Act and the 2021 American Rescue Plan Act approved $400 billion in federal funds to cover Covid testing, contract tracing, vaccines, and paid sick leave. Covid treatments, however, remain subject to insurance plans and patient responsibility.

The legislators did address flaws in the ACA. According to the Kaiser Family Foundation (KFF), the Rescue Plan expanded ACA Marketplace subsidies for people earning between 100 percent and 400 percent of the Federal Poverty Level. The subsidy increase lasts through 2022, meant to expire as Covid relents. It's temporary and does not help ACA patients long-term.

The Rescue Plan also extended eligibility for ACA subsidies to people making more than 400 percent of poverty.

Kaiser estimated that before the law, about eight million people were paying full-price for ACA coverage or held insurance plans purchased outside the ACA marketplace, most often because their incomes were too high to qualify for subsidies.

By expanding eligibility for Marketplace subsidies to the people earning above 400 percent of poverty, said KFF, "the law flattens the ACA's subsidy cliff and lowers premiums for virtually everyone already eligible for Marketplace subsidies." The benefit phases out at higher incomes for the higher premium plans. Even if short-lived, increased subsidies mean hard-pressed people can afford plans with lower deductibles, which translates into less medical debt.

As we publish this book in autumn 2021, Congress is prepared to pass a bipartisan $1.2 trillion Infrastructure Investment and Jobs Act. This bill includes $15 billion to replace lead water pipes in rural areas and low-income communities, which will reduce incidences of lead-induced diseases and related medical bills. This is "upstream thinking" for a healthy country.

Congress is trying to pass the Democrat's $3.5 trillion budget reconciliation bill, the Build Back Better Act, which has been whittled down by two "moderate" Democrat senators to about $2 trillion. The bill has as many progressive polices as the moderates will allow. Under Senate rules, the budget bill needs a basic one-vote majority vote to pass. The two bills, if enacted together as planned, represent the largest investment in economic development by the U.S. government since the New Deal in the Great Depression.

The infrastructure and jobs bill with the budget reconciliation bill, if passed, may improve the quality, accessibility and overall affordability of our healthcare system in the USA. Could be a big deal.

> The Build Back Better Act and the infrastructure bill, if passed, may improve the quality, accessibility and overall affordability of our healthcare system.

A two-year expansion of ACA premium subsidies could become permanent. Expanded subsidies could extend to families that before were ineligible if a family member had workplace health insurance. That would no longer matter in the ACA Marketplace. The plan would increase financial incentives for those states not yet using the ACA to expand Medicaid coverage.

Women of child-bearing age could get a parcel of "Momnibus" provisions, most with past bipartisan support, that aim to decrease maternal morbidity and mortality. Coverage for postpartum care could increase from 60 days to 12 months for women with Medicaid coverage, if their state allows.

Separately, President Biden has directed related federal agencies to reexamine Medicaid eligibility requirements and waivers, such as work rules, that have limited enrollment and care coverage.

These and other measure to improve the Affordable Care Act, of course, do not alter the fact that the ACA is still essentially a bundle of health insurance reform to get more people insured. The social benefit is people having affordable medical bills, but the ACA does not fundamentally change the underlying structure of how we finance healthcare — the structure that produces medical debt.

Regulate Insurance and Drug Prices

Can we reduce U.S. healthcare costs by regulating the profits of insurance and pharmaceutical companies? The advocates of "free market" economies oppose all limits on profits. Since we remain a capitalist nation, old-style price controls are unlikely.

Factually, industry regulation already is in effect in our country. Some would prefer less or no regulation, but in this moment for our nation, more regulation looks likely.

Insurance and pharmaceutical price reform is a Sisyphean task. The healthcare industry, including the hospital conglomerates and physicians, resists changes. Money keeps things the way they are.

A triumvirate of Big Insurance, Big Pharma and Big Hospitals benefit from the healthcare system as it is. I believe they mostly are concerned about how "the other" leg of the tripod is charging too much, thereby making it harder for them to charge more for their own big slice of the healthcare pie.

Robert Goff voiced his wisdom on hospitals and their system of profit margins over care missions. Let me look closer at two other so-called "bad boys" in healthcare costs — insurance companies and pharmaceutical companies.

U.S. health insurance corporate profits are booming. Bob Herman at Axios found that the five largest health insurers (UnitedHealthcare, CVS Health with subsidiary Aetna, Cigna, Anthem Blue Cross Blue Shield, Humana) together reported gross revenues of $786 billion for all 2019. Statista reported net profit for the Big Five rose to $8.4 billion in the second quarter of 2019, still higher a year later in 2Q 2020 (in pandemic) to $12.7 billion. Health insurance is a robust industry with healthy margins.

> A triumvirate of Big Insurance, Big Pharma and Big Hospitals benefits from the healthcare system as it is.

In an NPR interview, Herman said that since the ACA began, the cumulative salaries of insurance and pharma CEOs tallied $9.8 billion. One exec took home in excess of $900 million.

You might think all of this quality brainpower would make great allies for reformers trying to bring about financial reforms to relieve the burdens carried by folks like you and me. Not so. No motivation. Herman said executives are not paid to slow spending. Much of their pay is in stock and in stock options. "Their incentive is to do whatever it takes to make that stock go up." Stock prices drive drug prices, not that thin sliver of profits going for research.

Raising prices to lift stock values is the opposite of what we need to heal our broken system. Why not try to lower prices, eliminate unnecessary care and drugs, and coordinate care better? In my view, none of the Republican and Democratic proposals really address the core causes of rising costs in our healthcare system.

An intriguing development is "health insurance on demand." Pioneering the idea is a startup in Minneapolis called Bind Benefits.

The argument that high drug prices pay for all the R&D is a 'blatant fraud.' What's really driving up drug prices are stock buybacks and dividends.

Backed by UnitedHealthcare and partners, Bind uses data analytics to offer health consumers "only the coverage they need, when they need it, without narrowing their network."

On-demand insurance is said to be more affordable. Without high deductibles, Bind covers preventive care, primary and specialty care, urgent care, emergency care, hospital care, chronic care, and "pharmacy needs." Beyond its core package, Bind offers coverage as needed, like for cancer or pregnancy. On-demand insurance is a new model that may be a viable way to reduce medical debt

Bind has offered on-demand insurance only to self-funded companies plans, but the venture is expanding. *The Minneapolis Star-Tribune* and *Twin Cities Business* reported in 2020 that Bind had raised $105 million to launch fully insured health plans in dozens of states by 2021, including Florida. Texas, Virginia, Ohio, and Wisconsin. (*Covid interruptus.*)

Bind founding CEO Tony Martin told *FierceHealthcare* in 2021, "Healthcare leaders should understand and appreciate the power of better health insurance design. It's a critical part of the foundation needed to successfully address health disparities."

This leads me to the pharmaceutical industry.

Among all of the "out-of-control" health care sectors, the most widely attacked is the drug industry.

Why the outrage?

Eric Reguly, European Bureau Chief for *The Globe and Mail,* wrote a scathing article, "Rx for Excess: The truth behind big pharma spending," Reguly alleges that governments and consumers have been "brainwashed" into thinking double-digit price increases are necessary to fund all the world-class research and development programs, investing in inventing to make us healthier.

This rationale, apparently, condoned Gilead Sciences charging $84,000 for a 12-week course of treatment (at about $1,000 a pill) for Sovaldi, their antiviral therapeutic for Hepatitis C. *Médecins Sans Frontières* called the Gilead price "shocking," noting it would cost $227 billion to properly treat the 2.7 million Americans with Hep C, "let alone the rest of the world."

Reguly says the argument of "sumptuous prices for sumptuous R&D" is a "blatant fraud." What's really driving up drug prices are stock buybacks and dividends, he said, naming Valeant Pharmaceuticals' CEO, Michael Pearson, who in 2018 saw the valuations of his stock holdings and options swell to almost $3 billion.

The most blatant abuser may well be Purdue Pharma, the maker of OxyContin. Owned by the Sacker family, Purdue is the target of multi-billion dollar lawsuits for its central role in fostering the prescription opioid epidemic. The CDC blames opioid drugs for killing 500,000 Americans from overdoses in the two decades since 1999. rivaling the U.S. death toll for Covid of 750 million.

In August 2021, Dr. Richard Sackler told a bankruptcy court that Purdue would withhold billions from a negotiated legal settlement unless his family gets immunity for all current and future lawsuits. Will the Sackers keep their opioid billions?

Drug pricing reform is on the table. The reconciliation bill would cap out-of-pocket costs for prescriptions, increase insurance coverage for drugs (maybe eliminating the Medicare "donut hole"), increase fiscal liability of pharmaceutical makers, to reduce government's financial exposure, which means less taxpayer exposure.

Medicare at long last could negotiate drug prices directly with the drug manufacturers, the same as Medicaid and the Military Health System.

Medicare at long last could negotiate drug prices directly with manufacturers, the same as Medicaid and the Military Health System. It would help curb exponentially escalating drug prices for those in Medicare. Negotiated prices would index international drug prices. Americans would be able to buy FDA-approved drugs at prices close to those in Canada or Mexico. This may be life-saving for cancer patients and others with chronic disease now burdened by medical debt from costly medications they can't afford.

The bill would make drug manufacturers reimburse Medicare for single-use package drugs never used and discarded by providers. Unused medicines like cancer drugs cannot be recovered and must be disposed. CNBC estimated the annual loss at around $3 billion. This measure would plug one of the cost leaks in Medicare.

Seems to me that in today's rare political window, we actually can reduce U.S. healthcare costs by changing the marketplace where insurance and pharmaceutical companies conduct business.

The 'Public Option' and Medicare Expansion

We're hearing strong argument for adding a "Public Option" to the ACA, finally accepted as the law of the land. People propose lowering the age of eligibility from 65 years old to 60, 55 or 50. For this larger pool of Medicare recipients, same as now, supplemental insurance still would cover the 20 percent Medicare does not.

Private Medicare Part C Advantage plans would follow suite and open earlier enrollment. Age expansion would open a new market for Advantage plans that now serve about 40 percent those over age 65. Advantage plans cater to those who may not need or want full Medicare, let alone afford a supplemental. Such an age expansion of Medicare and Medicare Advantage plans would mean more older Americans would be less vulnerable to medical debt.

Two Trump era bills would have lowered the age of eligibility. They were introduced by Sen. Debbie Stabenow (D-MI), who saw Medicare starting at age 55, and Rep. Brian Higgins (D-NY), who saw it starting at age 50. Both bills relied upon marketplace subsidies and employer participation. Both promised earlier Medicare enrollment would not compete with commercial marketplace plans. Both bills failed to gain sufficient traction.

After the 2020 elections, the slim majority Democrats and some Republicans in the Senate and House committed in early 2021 to enactment of Medicare expansion. Partisan politics shifts promises. I hope it's been signed by President Biden when you read this.

Biden has called for lowering the age for Medicare to 60, but a lower age eligibility is not in the Build Back Better bill, yet as I write, the final smaller-scale bill is still being negotiated.

Another major expansion of Medicare could add dental, vision and hearing benefits to Parts A and. B. Under existing Medicare and most Advantage plans, these all have been out-of-pocket expenses. This would be a game-changer for seniors on fixed incomes.

An expansion of Medicare could add dental, vision and hearing benefits.

Funding for Medicare expansion is not finalized. Democrats offer such "payfors" as slightly raising corporate tax rates, but a key Democrat refuses. So, funding can come from better IRS tax enforcement and collections, from increased Medicare revenues through more enrollments by younger seniors; from huge Medicare cost savings by negotiated drug prices; and from greater "efficiencies" (which can be ephemeral." The backers of Medicare expansion also anticipate long-term economic growth that naturally generates more taxes to pay for the plan.

No matter what form Medicare expansion takes, if it ever does, detractors will deride it as "creeping socialism." For them, Medicare and Social Security are socialist schemes to rot out America's moral character and undermine personal responsibility. Even if true, few Americans will readily give it up. Have you ever given a dog a bone, even with scant meat on it, and tried to take it back?

As a point of reference, imagine America around 60 years ago when only 48 percent of all "senior citizens" had health insurance. About 35 percent of all seniors were living in poverty. Life expectancy was 66 years for men and 73 years for women. All that changed in 1965 with the passage of Medicare. Today, only two percent of us over age 65 live without healthcare coverage. Better, poverty among those age 65 and older has been reduced by two-thirds!

Now imagine people at age 50 enjoying such improvements in their life and health. Picture an America in which all elders enjoy the benefits of Medicare, with little or no medical debt.

Will bipartisan Medicare expansion pass the House and Senate? Will any Republicans vote to end medical debt for seniors?

And I must ask: Is Medicare expansion the best solution for us? Do you prefer a more sweeping change?

'Medicare for All' Single-Payer Healthcare

A 2018 Reuters survey determined that 70 percent of Americans support "Medicare for All," the then-current title for single-payer healthcare, same as in all other industrialized nations. During the 2020 elections, polls showed the popular support for single payer had increased. Seems that more Americans than politicians support universal healthcare. Some favor keeping the 80 percent cap with the gap covered by commercial supplemental insurance.

If Medicare expansion to more senior ever becomes a routine part of American society, I wonder, will the younger generations be a tad envious? Will we hear howls of protest from younger, healthier taxpayers unwilling to pay for their ailing elders! Will they march on Washington? Will they instead demand Medicare, too?

Reuters quoted Larry Levitt, the senior vice president for health reform at the Kaiser Family Foundation, "The advantage of Medicare for All, which is much closer to how the rest of the world provides health care to their residents, is that you can achieve universal health care at a lower cost."

Washington consultant Joel Segal, who co-wrote the language in the Affordable Care Act, earlier helped draft HR 676, "Expanded and Improved Medicare For All" — introduced in 2003 by the late Rep. John Conyers (D-MI) with 38 cosponsors. Segal recently told me the three main advantages of that single-payer solution:

1. No out-of-pocket costs.

2. No hospital or physician bills to pay.

3. No more medical debt.

Patients, physicians and hospitals would make decisions based on the need to generate health, not the need of insurance companies and medical providers in business to generate profits.

Under HR 676, healthcare would have been publicly financed, privately operated. This is different than the "socialized" national health system in England, Segal said, not like what we have in America at the troubled VA, "where government itself owns and operates the healthcare system."

Our health would stop being a profit center for corporations.

He added, "As in Medicare now, you show your government card, get care and go home. Unlike Medicare now, you need not worry about your 20 percent or bill collectors."

The proposal would have cut the 12 percent rate of uninsured people to zero. Everybody would be enrolled into one plan without deductibles or co-payments. Unlike with Medicare for seniors, all Americans would be fully covered from birth to grave.

People could buy supplemental private insurance, if they wish, Segal said, but other form of private health coverage would vanish. Our health would stop being a profit center for corporations

Most existing public programs as they exist today — including Medicare, Medicaid, and CHIP — would be subsumed into the new plan. Healthcare financing would shift away from households and employers to the federal government. Well, HR 676 failed.

Flash forward to 2019. The bill was revised with more details, renumbered HR 1384, renamed the "United States National Health

Care Act," and introduced in the 116th Congress by Rep. Pamela Jayapal (D-WA). The bill garnered 116 cosponsors in the House and support from almost half the congressional Democrats.

Naturally, the proposal had enemies. Beyond the ideological or morality issues in conservative quarters, critics raised the specter of cost. The Mercator Center in Virginia (Koch-funded) projected a $32.6 trillion increase in federal spending over ten years.

Answering critics was Sen. Bernie Sanders (D-VT), a cosponsor. He said, "If every major country on earth can guarantee health care to all and achieve better health outcomes while spending substantially less per capita than we do, it is absurd for anyone to suggest that the United States cannot do the same."

The bill failed to win passage during the Trump administration. Three months after the inauguration of the Biden administration, Jayapal introduced a refined version, HR 1976, the "Medicare for All Act of 2021," All attempts failed to include the resolution in the Rescue Act or reconciliation bill. Biden and moderate Democrats do not support it. Single-payer is a popular but elusive vision.

Healthcare as a Human Right

Could universal health care for every person at every age cost less and save money? That depends on whom you ask.

Physicians for a National Health Plan estimate a national health insurance program would save at least $150 billion annually on just paperwork alone. Under private insurance today, they argue, more than 25 percent of every health care dollar earned by the insurance companies goes not for claims but for marketing, billing, utilization review, and duplication (what some simply call "waste").

The Peterson-Kaiser *Health System Tracker* reported that other wealthy countries, on average, spend half as much per person on healthcare as the USA. This means that $10,000 in care charges here are $5,000 there. Anybody with a capitalist bent ought to love a solution that costs less and saves money, but I guess that depends on the capitalist and the situation.

Universal healthcare could offer a valuable public side-benefit: Equity in health care delivery. If single-payer universal healthcare is constructed in a way that my doctor is certifiably as good as your doctor, if our treatments are the same quality as yours, then we both have better health outcomes and quality of life. We do not compete for care. The system can focus on health not finance.

Single payer is a moral issue because all citizens deserve equal access to quality health care.

In Canada's single-payer system, reported *Newsweek*, "Medicine is not a commodity to be sold to the highest bidder, but a right that must be distributed equitably to one and all, and (like the Canadian character) ferociously egalitarian, but thrifty at the same time."

Why do we Americans resist such a sensible, moral social value? Seems this is where Americans reveal a form of Stockholm Syndrome. As the lifelong captives of "the system," we love our captors. We believe down is up.

For me, single payer is a moral issue because all citizens deserve equal access to quality health care. Does that turn me and other advocates of fairness into something un-American — a socialist? Really? Forget about labels. Ask what's right. We Americans need to take a moral stand that health is a basic human right. Biden has said he believes healthcare is a human right. Will he uphold his? I want our country to join the ranks of other enlightened nations.

The American Medical Debt Commission

I favor America no longer being a healthcare have-not nation. To get there, I'm learning how to think outside my box, thanks to conversations with people like Joel Segal. Hearing him tell about his private struggles with medical debt, as we explored our thoughts on healthcare in America, I had an "Aha!" moment.

It's one thing to begin a charity that forgives medical debt, I saw, yet it's something else entirely to grasp to change the laws governing medical debt. Joel has been drafting laws for years. He has shaped public policy in practical ways that affect our daily lives. His efforts made me realize that RIP has been playing too small.

Showing me what's possible, days after we met, Joel drafted the "The American Medical Debt Commission Act." Here's his text:

> Congress shall establish an independent bipartisan Medical Debt Commission that provides factual information on an annual basis to Congress and the general public about the medical debt crisis in America. A 25-member commission, chosen by the House Energy and Commerce Committee, would represent physicians, academics, hospital administrators, civil society organizations, local and state elected officials, foundations, think tanks, universities, medical debt experts, and the patients impacted by medical debt.

> The Commission would convene four times a year and publish an annual report about America's medical debt crisis, available for download at the website of the Centers for Medicare & Medicaid Services. The report would offer Commission recommendations on how to address the medical debt crisis with the broadest possible spectrum of solutions, based on best practices, aimed at ending the medical debt crisis in America.

At least once a year, Commission members would appear before the House committee to testify in public about the status of the U.S. medical debt crisis, reporting facts and results from the various attempted solutions addressing U.S. medical debt.

Joel could rapidly draft such a bill because he knows how. His mastery of the legislative process sparked in me a vision of the bold and audacious world in which I want to live — where we go beyond complaining about medical debt to actually ending it.

Committing to End Medical Debt

A this book publishes in October 2021, RIP has forgiven more than $5 billion in medical debt for individuals and families. That's laudable, a solid start, but let us not delude ourselves. We're only "sweeping up after the parade."

I'm convinced our deeper social purpose is awakening America to the problem of medical debt and galvanizing us into action. This book, I believe, contributes to that awakening.

Most Americans know our current healthcare system is broken. Despite the tired old bleat, "We can't afford it," most of us Americans want quality healthcare service for ourselves and our families with no more medical debt, nor the hardship debt creates.

We Americans already cough up enough in taxes to support the protections provided to us by our military, our police, and our fire departments. The same willingness to be taxed needs to happen for the protection of our health, physical and financial. We're spending as much or more for the current healthcare system.

We accept the tax burden for Medicare and Social Security, even if we grumble about it. When we get older and depend on Medicare and Social Security, we feel deeply grateful that we and others had the good sense and personal responsibility to pay those taxes.

Can enough of us educate ourselves out of fearful hopelessness, investigate our healthcare alternatives and choose more sensible solutions? Can enough of us accept that humane universal healthcare, based upon the experience of other nations, actually will cost us less money than we pay for the current system?

Hippocrates wrote, "Before you heal someone, ask him [*sic*] if he's willing to give up the things that made him sick." Medical debt makes far too many of us Americans sick and poor. Are we willing to give it up?

To realize America's founding promise of "Life, liberty, and the pursuit of happiness," let's note the order these words appear. Life, which relies on health, comes first. Without good health, liberty has little value, and the pursuit of happiness is meaningless. So, however we vote, America's health is on the ballot.

> Can enough of us educate ourselves out of fearful hopelessness, investigate our healthcare alternatives and choose more sensible solutions?

"If you have your health, you have everything," goes the saying. Let's stop depriving ourselves of that everything.

End medical debt.

Alone we can do so little;
together we can do so much

— HELEN KELLER

CHAPTER 13

A Meeting of Minds

Jerry Ashton, Robert E. Goff, Craig Antico

The three distinct authors have now shared their knowledge and views in 12 separate chapters. They offered real-world expertise in debt collections and hospital administration. Despite their diverse politics — progressive, moderate and conservative — they somehow united in 2014 to co-found RIP Medical Debt, a charity that to date has abolished $5.1 billion in unpayable healthcare bills.

Each author has updated and expanded what he originally wrote for the 2018 edition of *End Medical Debt.* When they chose together to publish a revised 2021 Covid recovery edition, they decided to add a final chapter with the three speaking together about Covid and our prospects for changing the healthcare delivery system.

Below is their conversation, covering new ground — transcribed and edited, curated into subhead sections for continuity. Notice the way they respond to one another's thoughts. Their interplay distills for me how their meeting of minds proved so dynamic in launching a movement to end medical debt in America.

— Judah Freed, editor

Covid Medical Debt

Editor: What are your thoughts about the condition of medical debt in the USA since the advent of Covid-19? For starters, are there any reliable estimates on the total amount of medical debt the pandemic may generate this year and in coming years?

Craig Antico: I can report numbers forecasted by the insurance companies. I figure they pretty much know what's going to be the patient's responsibility. Their actuarial assumption was that we have a 10 percent infection rate, as opposed to a 20 percent infection rate. At that rate, the estimate was $10 billion of Covid debt by June 2021. The estimate is likely high. We've had a lower infection rate, but that forecast was made before Delta, so it's too soon to know.

Jerry Ashton: Frankly, I'm horrified that the United States is approaching 45 million cases and 750,000 deaths from Covid and its variants. I'm upset most of the cases and deaths lately are among people who are not vaccinated. I'm upset our nation is not talking about all the people being harmed and suffering from the Covid care bills that will result in medical debt.

Robert Goff: With Covid debt, what we're seeing is the best and the worst. What puts this into the "best" category is that a number of hospitals put their collection activities on hold because of Covid, which is obviously positive. I'd like to believe the economic pressure that Covid has brought to so many, too many, has actually caused hospitals to wake up to the pressure their billing and debt collection practices add to individuals already under financial stress. I want to believe we're seeing humanitarian considerations prevail.

Lately, we're seeing an uptick in hospitals and others pursuing collections. It's because money was made available through federal stimulus funds, so collectors believe more people have money to pay off their debts.

In the "worst" category, we're seeing the usual exploitations of the system. I'm thinking of the New York physician, in Westchester County, I believe, who with county permission did Covid testing in parking lots. That was wonderful, but he tested for a broad range of things that just were not necessary. He was bilking huge amounts of money from insurance companies. When insurance started denying his claims, he started billing the patients.

The other thing we're seeing is typical inefficiencies, not nefarious, just plain old stupidity in the system's inability to bill properly. You have people being billed for Covid testing, people found to have Covid because they were tested, but Covid was not on the diagnosis, so all their treatments have not been covered by federal funds.

Craig: And Covid debt goes to those same groups of poor people who get most of the medical bills and have most of the medical debt. They live just above two times the poverty level, or maybe three and a half times the poverty level. They are the ones most getting hurt. The elderly and lowest wage workers are getting hurt. The people on the front lines who earn the least but have the most exposure to Covid are getting hurt.

> I'm upset our nation is not talking about all the people suffering from Covid care bills that will result in medical debt.
>
> — *Jerry Ashton*

Another factor is that fewer hospitals are selling their Medicare debt [unpaid balances after Medicare pays 80 percent]. If they don't sell their Medicare debt, then RIP can't access it for debt forgiveness. It's an inordinate amount of debt, billions a year.

Covid debt also is generated by hospitals from self-pay patients for the balance after insurance. From RIP, we know people of color have a very high percentage of medical debt on their credit reports, as compared to white people. The first waves of Covid in 2020 hit people of color the hardest. That's not true with Delta, where mostly unvaccinated and more affluent white people are getting sick.

Robert: If a person with Covid has no insurance, the best thing for them may be that the federal government is stepping up to pay the bills, which comes from all of us taxpayers.

If an older person with Covid is on Medicare, and if they have a good supplemental plan, medical bills are unlikely, assuming they stay in-network with Medicare. If they don't have a supplemental plan, they must self-pay that other 20 percent. A low-end plan may leave bills. too. Any unpaid bills become medical debt.

Some self-insured companies are saying that if an employee gets a Covid diagnosis, their group insurance will pick up 100 percent of the bills. That's very good, but it leaves out people who work where employers are not so generous. Some have gaps in their coverage if they get ill from Covid, and their care will produce high bills. There is a question if these bills will be paid by the government, like those with no insurance. If not, if they cannot pay, that's still more medical debt from Covid that goes into collections.

Covid Debt Collections

Jerry: Debt collection is one of the few economic sectors helped by Covid. There's increased employment in our old industry. The agencies are piling on employees, I understand, and they're making all kinds of money. Now, what do you think about that?

Craig: The interesting thing here is that after the pandemic first struck and the government began picking up the tab for Covid care, there were still old medical bills in collection.

Collections slowed when Covid began and agency offices closed. Collectors working in boiler rooms did not want to be in each other's faces. Making collections calls is something that can be done from home, so agencies pushed out office workers to be home workers. In time, boiler rooms were going at full steam, but now from collector's living rooms.

That shift was a big disruptor, and that's part of the reason why debt collections went down at first. Another reason was the practical collectability of any account with so many people out of work.

A bigger reason was sensitivity about going after people when they are down and even ill. That makes sense. It's similar to what happens when a tornado or a hurricane hits. They always stop all collections in that locale for awhile.

> ## Collections slowed when Covid began and agency offices closed. Collectors working in boiler rooms did not want to be in each other's faces.
>
> *— Craig Antico*

The debt industry couldn't stop all collections during Covid, not if collectors at home were to keep their jobs. But some places were forced to stop. Some states would not allow collections, especially for health care bills. New York State cut off all collections, just cut it off. The governor ordered hospital not to enable legal collections, not to file suits on overdue accounts, which I think is pretty amazing! The University of Virginia completely stopped placing any bills with collection agencies, and that's where they collect must of their money to run the university, so... wow!

Covid Economic Impacts

Editor: How is Covid medical debt tied to the condition of the whole economy? We've had a big downturn. When enough of us got vaccinated, the economy began to rebound. What can you say about the economy recovering from the pandemic?

Craig: One thing I find interesting is that in the downturn of the economy from Covid, with so many people losing their jobs, I really expected to see a tremendous uptick in the number of uninsured, and that's not what was happening.

One reason may be because ACA Marketplace plans are not tied to an employer. That's big. This is one of the first times we're able to see how the safety net of the ACA is really helping people to weather the storms of a recession. As a result, my perspective on healthcare deserts and debt mountains has changed dramatically. I'm actually kind of encouraged by some of the things I'm seeing,

Jerry: I'd like to compliment Craig for seeing these things and for rethinking his views. I'm probably becoming even more militant than before Covid. The fact is that we have a perfect storm to test every part of our healthcare system. Whether it fragments, fractures or breaks apart, or gets healthier, we'll have to see.

I think that all this tragedy gives us a really great chance to help people understand the healthcare system better, especially from our viewpoint of eliminating medical debt.

Craig: Well, that may really depend on whether Biden can get through Congress what he wants to do. It's proving difficult with such a slim majority in both houses, especially in the Senate, to push through legislation and change the law.

There was a lot of support in 2020 for a "Medicare for All" type of a system, but I don't think we're going to see it now, Biden said he won't support it. The insurance system stays in place.

I do believe we'll see a way for more people to have insurance. Right now, about 10 percent of all Americans don't have insurance. If Medicare and Medicaid expansion happens, it's conceivable at best it we'll get to the equivalent of what we call "full employment" — less than five percent unemployment. If we get to something like "full insurance," we'd still have five percent uninsured, and they likely will have medical debt.

More people than that will still be underinsured. The bad thing is that deductibles are going to be too high for most people, because costs for care are not coming down. We see it showing up as medical debt, where it doesn't matter if a person had insurance or not.

> Covid is one of the first times we're able to see how the safety net of the ACA is really helping people to weather the storms of a recession.
>
> — *Craig Antico*

Robert: We keep forgetting, as a society, that the price of health insurance is dictated by the cost of delivering care services. Everybody wants to lower the very high cost of health insurance, or make it vanish, but nobody is addressing *why* the cost of care is as high as it is.

Biden put in place a plan for mass immunizations, which has let people go back to work. He's spent money to help people who lost their jobs, stimulating the economy. There's money for hospitals to keep them from going under, but is it wasted? In reality, there's nothing in the plans before Congress that fundamentally addresses the cost drivers of healthcare or the infrastructure of healthcare delivery. Both need to change.

Jerry: We don't know certain things. We don't know what new laws will get through Congress. We don't know how pharmaceutical companies will use all the money pouring it into their bottom lines from government for Covid testing, vaccinations and therapeutics. How much of that money will go for developing drugs to sell to the American public at high prices? How much of the money will go for marketing and slick advertising?

Holistic Health Care

Editor: How about alternatives to costly medical practice?

Robert: Nothing yet really makes health itself a central part of healthcare delivery. There's little acceptance of a holistic approach to care. Focusing on better health is the most reliable and least used way to bring down the costs of care. Our health is where personal responsibility matters most.

Craig: Yes, patients play a big role in this. They need to discuss with their physicians all aspects of treatment plans, not just clinical care, but its economics.

> ## Our health is where personal responsibility matters most.
>
> — *Robert E. Goff*

Physicians can and should participate in guiding patients to affordable in-network care for their community. Doing it requires their time to gain familiarity with quality providers in the local narrow network. How can they afford the time for this?

The physician has an ethical obligation to care for patients clinically as well as to care for the patients' overall financial health. A holistic view is that undue stress opens patients to disease. That level of care is only going to happen if the patient and physician work together.

Jerry: I like the physician being accountable for the financial health of a patient. Yes, absolutely. If the patient gets sick, in some cultures, the doctor has to pay.

Robert: If you look at the history of managed care, it really started in ancient China. The warlords would say to the physician. I will pay you, not for the people you take care of sick, but the number of people who work in my field or go fight in my army. If they can't work or fight, they don't bring me value, so neither do you. You saw this thinking in China's early public health and personal hygiene activities.

Craig: The thing is that people really could be healthier, but the system doesn't support health like it should. Our overall health is the key determinant of whether or not we go to the doctor or hospital.

Robert: A better model is the idea of looking at the patient holistically, trying to wrap around that person the full range of care services they need for health. If patient requirements extend beyond the specific resources of an institution, a holistic approach would not stop at the institution's door.

> A better model is the idea of looking at the patient holistically, trying to wrap around that person the full range of care services they need for health.
>
> — Robert E. Goff

A hospital or private practice that actually works to wrap patients in clinical services needs reliable access to all community resources, like public health, social services, mental health, behavioral health. Addressing the needs of the whole person means that healthcare does not stop at restoration from illness or injury, but pays attention to the circumstances that gave rise to the episode itself.

> We face a challenge in getting the healthcare industry to treat the patient as a whole human being, not just a body with fixable parts moving along some assembly line.
>
> — *Jerry Ashton*

To reduce the medical costs of a homeless person, for instance, you first need to create a home situation. A lot of upstream issues have to do with the quality of the housing, the quality of food, knowledge and understanding of personal hygiene and mental health issues. These are not now addressed in the clinical setting. I'm talking about a broader approach of wrapping care around a person.

Craig: To do that, health records systems can be more intertwined with insurance records, so physicians and patients know up front what care is or is not covered. Using a secure navigator of some sort, like a GPS for care providers, patients could actually be told quickly where to go in-network for their ailments. Fewer may go out-of-network or just go to the ER.

Robert: Broader than clinical care is the physician training. Medical care now is all about a diagnosis and how to treat it. If I'm a physician, my game plan is treating that clinical diagnosis in my realm of expertise, so I get the billing, or my employer gets the billing. Instead, it should be all about helping the whole person by bringing in community resources.

Jerry: I agree, but the argument against the holistic approach is that it will increase costs even higher.

Robert: Actually, in the world of end-stage renal disease, people on dialysis who maintain a tight diet have been shown to reduce the number of treatments they need to maintain health. Their personal responsibility improves their quality of life and decreases costs.

Jerry: So it's okay for me to be holistic and healthy as long as I'm not living in a food desert or transportation desert, or I'm not under so many medical bills that I can't afford to buy good groceries over junk groceries. We face a big challenge getting the healthcare industry to treat the patient as a full human being, not just a body with fixable parts moving along some assembly line.

Robert: This is the failure of the healthcare system to be a health promotion system. Do you design a system based on better health or on treating illness and injury? If you go after good health, you must address what Jerry mentioned to help people stay healthy.

This extends to health factors like water, air and land pollution. A hospital in New York City, close to a highway, treats an awful lot of asthma cases that may be related to exhaust fumes coming off that highway. Where do you go to address this cost driver?

Jerry: That's a matter of public policy. If the policy of that city is that they don't give a damn what people downstream say about the pollution, then no money is allocated to take care of such things. In politics, without public pressure, there is no intervention.

Who Pays for Care?

Craig: Are you talking about government or non-governmental intervention? Can the private sector help to change upstream health factors? Who provides the funds? Are you talking about donors? Years ago, United Way had people give one percent of their income, which supported a tremendous amount of social services in the community. A lot of times, business would match it. That federated fundraising model worked for a long time. It used to be that 60 percent of all individual donations went to churches, which used much of it for community social services. Now it's only 30 percent. That federated fundraising system is gone.

What we see at RIP today, as a private charity, is that people generously support other people doing local medical debt relief campaigns. Otherwise, that debt remains on the books and in collections. Worse, I know from RIP that medical debt is way too unfairly distributed to people that can barely afford it. Is there any way, without becoming a socialist country, without forcing people into it, to spread the costs of care across more people?

> # Is there any way, without becoming a socialist country, to spread the costs of care across more people?
>
> — *Craig Antico*

Jerry: My answer, Craig, is that the so-called "government handout" is really us handing out to us.

The main problem is that today's tax structure for spreading the pain doesn't work fairly. If you're spreading the pain with one percent for you and for me, us working stiffs, and one percent for somebody who has $500 million, is that fair?

This is where ethics and morality come in. Do we take care of our brothers, or do we only pay lip service to it?

Once upon a time, the wealthy were willing to pay their fair share, same as some of the wealthiest today say they'd gladly pay higher taxes. But too many wealthy people are unwilling to pay their fair share, or they don't want to pay any taxes at all.

Without everybody paying their fair share, there's not enough money or no money to lesson the pain at the lower levels of society. If you live at that lower level, even if you have income, you are as close to being in hardship as anybody now, and that's not right. It's only because some people are not paying their fair share.

Robert: We have interesting examples of a community doing that. The Amish took themselves out of governmental social systems, but they still meet the social and medical needs of their community. The Mennonite community, from what I gather, does not participate in Social Security, Medicare or Medicaid. All medical bills are paid by the community on behalf of the membership. I believe members pay a percent of their income.

As for doing something like this on a national level, the closest we can come to universal distribution of the costs for providing care is through tax policy. There's no other means.

Objectives and Incentives

Editor: Is it possible that we can change public opinion enough to change the healthcare system's structure, so it stops generating medical debt? Changes in the ACA only changed the way insurance pays care providers for services rendered.

Craig: There has to be an alignment of objectives and incentives. In term of restructuring health insurance, for example, if there were fewer narrow networks, or no narrow network, we would have 20 percent less debt on people's back for out-of-network bills. Well, the healthcare and insurance companies don't want that. It may reduce patient debt but it would increase their business costs.

If we required by law lower insurance premiums, it could lower people's costs below the 15 percent of income most of us now pay for premiums, but that won't lower care delivery costs, so the system will just come up with some other way to cost shift.

We need to aligned our goals here, but I don't know how we can align insurance companies with individuals on this.

Robert: Remember that health insurance is a function of what care costs. Health insurance costs what it costs because of what it costs to buy care services. The fact is, care costs have gone up.

This is why employee plans have decreased coverage, increased co-pays, or increased payroll deductions. If the employers would be willing to pay more, employees would better covered, but it reduces profitability, maybe to the point of losing the business.

So, you have to address the bottom-line issue. Why does it cost what it costs? Should it cost that? Is there a way of delivering better medical care that costs less?

This question is not addressed by Affordable Care Act insurance reforms. Insurance companies are treated like a public utility with a limit on profitability. The ACA requires they spend 80 to 85 percent of the premiums for care reimbursement. If the insurance company spends more, the cost comes out of their coffers. If they spend less, the surplus is rebated to the policy holder. So, blaming insurance company profits, in this case, is really misdirected.

The ACA did make health insurance more affordable, but it did not change the care delivery system itself, or reduce its costs, and those costs are what drive the price of insurance coverage.

Structural System Changes

Jerry: Trying to make real structural changes in the healthcare delivery system looks nearly impossible right now. I doubt America has the political will.

Robert: You're talking about doing a massive amount of public education. There's so much distrust now in all parts of the system, especially drug companies, insurance companies, and the hospital industry. That distrust runs deep.

And even if we commit to changing popular opinion, who is going to organize that big public education effort? What does the campaign advocate in practical terms, and what is the outcome of that education going to be?

Let's suppose, for fun, that you can plan the ideal health delivery system for a community, and you figure out a fair way to finance it. The world fast comes up with reasons why you should not do it. It would mean the change or closure of a beloved facility. People do not want to change a care system they know, even if it's wasteful or doesn't work, Change is scary.

Years ago, a very fine physician I know ran a state commission on improving maternity services in the State of New York. The commission came up with a master plan that included closing down a number of ineffective and lower quality maternity units. The outcry against him was incredible. He even had death threats. The goal of the plan, of course, was improving the quality of maternity care, which is exactly what ended up happening. When the dust settled, quality did go up, but some hospitals lost their maternity departments. Those communities believe they lost something of value.

> Let's suppose that you can plan the ideal health delivery system for a community, and you figure out a fair way to finance it. The world fast comes up with reasons why you should not do it.
>
> — *Robert E. Goff*

Robert: Some rural and urban communities have looked at how to serve people outside the box of their existing care delivery infrastructure, which is largely brick and mortar. We used to think retail meant brick and mortar stores. Online shopping showed us new possibilities.

Now we're seeing the same thing for hospitals in small communities. Apart from sudden demand for beds from the Covid surges, most small rural hospitals do not have ongoing a high volume of patients. They lack the usage to support increasing their care capacity, like buying the latest digital imaging technology. They cannot support a whole lot of sophistication in medical care, such as the very latest advances in oncology.

It doesn't help anybody to create a false impression that all people can receive the best possible care in their community when that's practically impossible. Another care delivery model is necessary.

Editor: Far easier said than done. Have any specifics in mind?

Robert: Well, one thing that's advanced nicely during Covid is telemedicine. Whether or not it will continue after the pandemic is still unclear, but I hope it does.

> The problem is that the capital investment we have in the current costly infrastructure of healthcare sucks up all the dollars. It precludes us from starting with a blank slate, which is what we need to do.
>
> — *Robert E. Goff*

Telemedicine gives us the ability to deliver healthcare remotely, which is terrific. There are limitations when not physically present, of course, but telemedicine lets us add life-saving sophistication to care delivery. In Israel, for example, most recovering Covid patients are discharged from the hospital quickly and sent home with a package of technology that lets the physician remotely monitor patients' vitals. That's not really possible in our country because we don't yet have universal internet service.

We need to look at care delivery in a different manner. I've seen presentations on the military developing the capability to deliver care services remotely in combat areas or behind the lines.

Increasing costs increases debt.
— *Craig Antico*

Mobile units with surgical robots can link by satellite to surgeons sitting thousands of miles away. That may save lives.

We could use such tech to give people in rural areas the quality care they need and deserve. It's going to require a different structure for medical care delivery. Telemedicine and remote monitoring help to reduce the number of expensive hospitals going underutilized, and it builds flexible emergency response capacity for crises, such as in pandemics and natural disasters.

Remote care also can help save lives in densely populated urban areas. If a person has an auto accident or acute episode, like a stroke, you might have three to six minutes to address the crisis. In busy traffic, like midtown or Harlem, you're probably not going to get an ambulance there in time. What can you do?

Could you integrate remote access, maybe with drones, operated by medics who deliver life support services until a patient can be transported by road or air to a medical facility? Widespread public training in basic first aid training and CPR could help save lives.

> If America is going to see any lasting change in the structure of financing healthcare delivery, we need to build a consensus on the need to change the basic system.
> We need to agree on a clear vision of what to do instead.
> — Jerry Ashton

Craig: That would save lives, but increasing costs increases debt, which may harm the lives being saved.

Robert: Again, we have to think outside the box. The problem is that the capital investment we have in the current costly infrastructure of healthcare sucks up all the dollars. It precludes us from starting with a blank slate, which is what we need to do.

Another piece we've learned from Covid is that we have the ability to open pop-up hospitals with hundreds of beds. This gives us an ability to shut down costly underutilized hospitals, knowing we have the ability to open hospitals as needed, like in a tornado or wildfire, instead of maintaining the high overhead of underutilized brick and mortar hospitals. If combined with quality telemedicine and mobile teams, this could help lead to reduced healthcare costs overall.

Craig: If you think about closing these facilities, from an employment standpoint, of the 168 million people employed in our nation, 14 percent work in healthcare. That's expected to go up. One reason it's hard to change the healthcare system structure is because it employs so many people.

Saving the millions of healthcare jobs keeps healthcare from changing. What are we going to do? If we eliminate, let's say, one-third of all the healthcare jobs as ineffective or as too costly, we may have a recession. After losing their jobs, unemployed people are the least able to buy insurance and pay their medical bills. This winds up increasing medical debt.

Jerry: If America is going to see lasting change in the structure of financing healthcare delivery, we need to change public opinion. We need to build consensus on the need to change the basic system. We need to agree on a clear vision of what to do instead.

Funding for this nationwide public education may have to come from the NGOs [non-governmental organizations], foundations and major donors. They still have a modicum of trust left in the country. They can help us do together what we cannot do alone.

Through our combine efforts, like in this book, we're helping to educate America about how to end medical debt for good.

*Hope lies in dreams, in imagination,
and in the courage of those who dare
to make dreams into reality.*

— JONAS SALK, MD

About the Authors

Jerry Ashton — Jerry is a four-decade veteran of the collections industry who rethought his career and profession after being inspired by his work in the Occupy Wall Street movement. He turned from debt collector to debt forgiver, which led him in 2014 to co-founding RIP Medical Debt.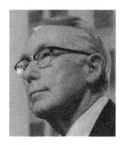
Achieving in 2020 his goal of RIP abolishing $1billion in medical debt, Jerry retired to RIP's board and founded LetsRethinkThis.com to address and solve other societal problems.

Robert E. Goff — With more than 45 years of experience in the healthcare industry, Robert E. Goff is a respected expert in care delivery, organization and financing. His career spans a range of leadership roles as a hospital administrator, managed care executive, consultant, regulator,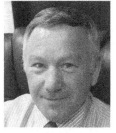
and association executive, retiring recently as the Executive Director and CEO of University Physicians Network, based in New York. A founding director of RIP Medical Debt, he serves on its Board.

Craig Antico — Before co-founding RIP, Craig ran companies that bought and collected debt for a profit. Today, he's a sought-after expert in debt forgiveness and identifying the people with debt causing hardship. He's been interviewed by such national media as *NBC Nightly News*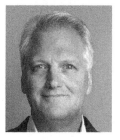
with Lester Holt, PBS Newshour, The Doctors, New York Times, and *Wall Street Journal. Town and Country* named him as a top forty Philanthropist of the Year. He is Emeritus on the RIP Board.

Forgiveness is not an occasional act,
it is a constant attitude.

— MARTIN LUTHER KING, JR.

RIP
ᴧEDICAL
DEBT

About RIP Medical Debt

RIP Medical Debt is a 501(c)(3) not-for-profit national charity based in New York, incorporated in 2014, which locates, buys and cancels unpayable medical bills for those burdened by financial hardship.

RIP to date has abolished more than $5 billion in medical debt nationwide by supporting local community debt relief campaigns, cancelling hospital bad debt and forgiving veteran medical debt.

RIP buys portfolios of unpayable medical billing accounts at near a penny on the dollar. A $100 donation can cancel $10,000 in debt, so the donors to RIP get "a lot of bang for the buck."

Surprised people who receive RIP debt relief are notified by mail in a golden envelope. These charitable gift have no tax consequences. Debt relief from RIP is a freely given random act of kindness.

For more information, visit RIPmedicaldebt.org

Even if you're on the right track,
you'll get run over if you just sit there.

— WILL ROGERS